Amazing Posture Facts

- In one study, participants were shown photos of two women—and the one with good posture was consistently judged younger and more attractive, even though she was older than the other and twenty pounds heavier.

- Poor posture is the primary cause of back pain—and can also be responsible for neck pain, leg pain, headaches, and other chronic physical symptoms.

- Good posture can improve breathing capacity and athletic performance.

- Your posture has a big impact on how others see you—and how you see yourself.

With *Posture, Get It Straight!* you can discover the dramatic and surprising benefits of improved posture—and take a stand for better health.

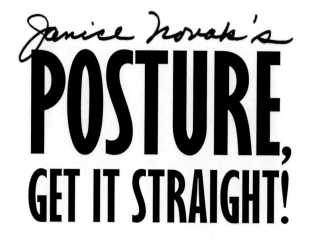

Janice Novak's
POSTURE, GET IT STRAIGHT!

Illustrations by Barbara A. Beshoar

Disclaimer:

As with all matters concerning health, the instructions, procedures, and advice in this book are in no way intended as a substitute for medical counseling. We strongly recommend you consult your doctor and physical therapist before beginning this or any exercise program. Only your physician knows your personal medical history and can advise you appropriately. The author and publisher cannot be help responsible for any results arising from use or application of the information in this book.

Ordering Information

To order the companion exercise DVD and/or non-latex resistance bands, go to www.ImproveYourPosture.com or call 1-952-949-9845.

Discounts available on this book and/or companion DVD, when ordered in quantity or for special sales.

Illustrations by Barbara A. Beshoar
Cover design and interior layout by Purpose Design

ISBN 13: 978-1-931945-62-2
ISBN 10: 1-931945-62-4

Library of Congress Catalog Number: 2006930349

Printed in the United States of America

First Printing: May 1999
Second Printing: August 2006

10 09 08 07 06   5 4 3 2 1

Expert Publishing, Inc.
14314 Thrush Street NW
Andover, MN 55304-3330
Andover,   1-877-755-4966
Minnesota www.expertpublishinginc.com

Dedication

I dedicate this book to my two beautiful daughters, Kate and Rachael. I am proud to say they are shining examples of young women who carry themselves with strength and confidence. They are the light of my life and they keep me on my toes.

Contents

Preface

I became interested in posture in my early twenties. When I was a teenager, I grew several inches over one summer. This made me taller than most of the girls my age and most of the boys as well. I didn't like that at all. As a result, I slumped on purpose so I would fit in better.

Then I reached my twenties and being tall suddenly wasn't so bad. But, unfortunately, a lot of damage was already done. I remember running into an old high school friend who showed me pictures taken at a high school party. I was shocked and horrified to see how slumped my upper back had become and how rounded my shoulders were. I knew I wasn't born this way and that I had done this to myself. So I set out to see if I could undo this damage. Was it possible to get my shoulders straight again? Was it possible to take that unsightly slump out of my upper back so my head wouldn't protrude so far forward? By trial and error, I found that not only was it possible, it wasn't even that difficult. This is the information I am so proud to share with you.

When I decided to put all this info in book form, my agent shopped it around to all the publishing houses in New York City. One of the publishers we contacted happened to be having a lot of trouble with his neck. When he read the chapter on the ABCs of Computer Comfort, he took my advice and re-arranged his computer screen, monitor, and computer chair. Within the first week of doing so, he discovered his neck and back felt much better. He was thrilled to find my advice worked so quickly and so well, and we were thrilled to find that he wanted to publish my book. What he liked best was the fact that the advice contained within was simple to implement. He didn't have to go out and buy new furniture. He just had to re-arrange the furniture he already had to make working at his computer infinitely more comfortable.

The beauty of this book lies in its simplicity. All of the tips, techniques and exercises are simple yet extremely effective.

I wrote this book for every male and female who thought it was impossible to correct his or her posture. I wanted everyone to see that no matter how bad their posture may be or how long they've had poor posture, it is never too late. You can improve your posture, and in the process not only look better, but also rid yourself of a whole array of common aches and pains. Improving posture is simply a matter of becoming aware of a few things, such as how you stand, sit, and move, then strengthening the muscles that have become too weak and stretching ones that have become too tight and overburdened. It is quite simple.

I am extremely grateful to all the people who have come through my work-shops for they have helped me perfect my program. Over the years they've told me which of my techniques and exercises helped them the most and which needed to be tweaked to become more user-friendly. Because of them, this is an extremely effective program that will have you standing straighter in no time at all.

Acknowledgements

I am eternally grateful to all of the wonderful teachers from whom I've had the privilege of learning. I'd like to thank all the people who've participated in my classes and workshops over the years. I've learned much from their questions and experiences. I'd also like to thank Mary Jo Sherwood for her professional experience and her help in bringing my program to many more people. She is a true friend and cherished colleague. She has undoubtedly helped make this a better book.

Part I

Standing Tall

What Good Posture Can Do for You

- *Do you think you would look better if you could just lose ten pounds?*
- *Are you plagued by back pain? A sore neck? Headaches?*
- *Have you been shocked by how rounded over you look in photographs?*
- *Do you think you look older than your years?*
- *Would you like to look ten years younger?*

If you answered yes to any of these questions, you can make a big difference in your health and your appearance by simply improving your posture.

When you were a child or a teen, was your mother always telling you to straighten up? She meant well, of course, but just straightening up is not the answer. When most people try to improve their posture, they jam their shoulders back, suck in their bellies, and stand stiff as soldiers. This is wrong not only because no one can sustain the position for more than a few seconds, but also because it does not align the body properly. The position looks and feels unnatural and uncomfortable.

For more than fifteen years, I have taught workshops to help people align their bodies quickly and naturally. My program is not a drug, surgical procedure, alternative therapy, elastic garment, or magic spell. Instead, it is a step-by-step alignment technique that will have you standing straighter instantly and will keep you standing straighter through a combination of stretching and strengthening exercises and practical tips for better posture. The results are both immediate and lasting.

I'm often asked, "After years of bad posture, is there any hope for me?" My answer is always an enthusiastic *yes*! No matter how bad your posture is at this moment, you can turn things around with little difficulty. You can start having better posture not in months, weeks, or even days, but in minutes. The One Minute To Better Posture technique will have you standing straighter immediately. The exercises will strengthen the muscles that support good posture. If you spend even a few minutes a day practicing the One Minute To Better Posture technique and some of the exercises, you'll see a big change in only five weeks.

If you are not currently happy with your posture, you have a lot of company. Bad posture is so common because many of us sit too much, exercise too little, and have habits like hanging our heads forward over our desks and always carrying heavy purses and briefcases on the same side of our bodies.

My program approaches posture improvement in three ways: alignment, a combination of stretching and strengthening exercises to maintain alignment, and small but powerful changes in everyday habits such as how you sit, sleep, and lift things. The tips, techniques, and exercises can easily be fit into your daily activities without having to set aside a special chunk of time. Learn the exercises and then do a few here and there throughout your day. In no time at all, you'll be reaping the many benefits of standing tall. For inspiration, let's start by taking a closer look at the benefits you'll reap.

Look Ten Pounds Thinner

Simply by standing straight, you will instantly slim your waistline by an inch or more. Check it out! Place a cloth measuring tape around your waist and assume your normal stance. Now lift up your rib cage slightly, as if a string attached to your breastbone were pulling it toward the ceiling. With your rib cage lifted slightly, see how much tighter you can pull the tape. You'll be pleasantly surprised.

The anatomical explanation for this seemingly magical change is that when the upper back slumps forward, it presses the rib cage down on the abdominal organs causing your midsection to widen and your belly to protrude more.

Look Ten Years Younger

A study in Louisville, Kentucky, showed how posture affects perceptions of age and beauty. Two women, both five foot four inches, one weighing 105 pounds and the other 125, were asked to put on leotards and cover their faces. Side view pictures were taken of each woman with normal and slumping posture.

Then sixty people were asked to look at the pictures and rate the women's appearances. When the women stood up straight, viewers consistently described them as younger and more attractive. In fact, the upright 125-pound woman was rated more favorably than the slumping 105-pound woman.

Nothing ages you faster than a shrinking, stooped posture. A strong, straight spine portrays youth and vigor. Slumping forward decreases your chest measurement, rounds and narrows your shoulders, and can decrease your height by as much as two inches.

If you ever had your height measured only to be told you are shorter than the last time you were measured, chances are you haven't actually shrunk. Most often it is that your spinal curves have become more exaggerated and that is what has caused the height loss. If your height difference was because of poor posture, there is great news! You can regain that lost height by practicing the One Minute To Better Posture technique in chapter three.

Radiate Confidence

Psychological studies have shown that a person with good posture exudes health, vitality, and confidence, while slouching signals insecurity, weakness, and self-doubt. Consciously or not, we tell the world a lot about our mental and emotional state by the way we stand, sit, move, and carry ourselves. In fact, posture is one of the first three things people notice about each other (the other two are hair and eyes).

Improving your posture can help you build self-esteem, radiate confidence and capability, interview well for jobs, and improve work performance (particularly in sales or business). Other people will see you with a new eye. Good posture shows the world you respect yourself. This commands respect from others.

Improve Your Athletic Performance and Decrease Chance of Injury

Because poor posture causes your joints to no longer fit together properly, when you work out or play sports, the chance that you will injure your neck, shoulder, upper back, lower back, hips, and knees is greatly increased. Good posture reduces the chance of injury, muscle strain, and aches; helps you move more easily, gracefully, and powerfully; and gives your lungs more room so you have a greater breathing capacity.

Prevent Back Pain

Most important, good posture can prevent a lifetime of annoying and painful back and neck problems. *Poor posture is the leading cause of back pain.*

The spine, or backbone, is the main supporting structure of the entire body. It is composed of twenty-four interlocking bones called vertebrae, which are stacked one upon the other. In between the vertebrae are disks. This is a delicate, finely balanced structure that can easily be injured. When posture is poor, the joints no longer fit together the way they're supposed to. If joints are poorly aligned, even common, everyday activities cause uneven wear and tear, resulting in friction, pain, irritation, and osteoarthritis.

When the spine is lined up correctly, the muscle groups that support it are in balance. When the slight natural curves in the spine become exaggerated, some muscles are put in a stretched position all day causing them to continually weaken. Other muscles are contracted all day and they become too tight and tense. Poor posture causes some muscles to overwork while others don't work at all. Gradually, the muscles lose their ability to support the body correctly, and posture grows even worse.

If the lower back arches too much, pressure on the joints and the nerves that pass between them can cause dull aches or stabbing, burning pain anywhere from the waist to the tip of the big toe. A head that hangs forward, even slightly, exaggerates the curve in the upper part of the spine and can cause chronic back pain, a stiff or sore neck, or tingling or numbness in the arms and hands. The head-forward position is also a common cause of tension headaches, the most common kind of headache.

Knowing the basics of good posture can make the difference between a healthy back and an aching one. When properly aligned, your body moves with ease and comfort. The muscles in the front and back of your body work together harmoniously. You will look better and feel better.

The goal of this book is not to have you stand in a stock-straight military posture, but to help ease you into a natural, relaxed alignment.

A Few Cautions Before You Begin
Exercise Precautions:

- Always consult an M.D. before doing any exercise program.

- Always warm up before doing any exercise. Warming up get your muscles ready for exercise by increasing their temperature and the flow of blood. A warm-up is especially important if you have been sitting all day or have been out in the cold. Before you do strengthening or resistance exercises (or aerobic activity or sports, for that matter), warm up. Gently, continuously move your arms and legs for five to ten minutes. An easy way to warm up is to walk in place. While you're walking, circle your shoulders forward and backward several times. Hunch your shoulders toward your ears, then press them away. Inhale deeply several times to expand your rib cage. Exhale deeply, too. Gently swing your arms by your sides, then from your sides to the ceiling. Slowly turn your chin toward your right shoulder, then your left, a few times.

- Never hold your breath. When you are concentrating on a new exercise, it is easy to forget to breathe. Holding your breath deprives your exercising muscles of oxygen. It can even give you a headache. If you tend to hold your breath, then count the repetitions out loud. You can't hold your breath when you are verbally counting.

- Relax! Only the muscles you are working should be tight. As you do the exercises, consciously relax your forehead and jaw. Don't furrow your brow or clench your teeth. Remember to drop your shoulders away from your ears.

- Stretch the muscles you have just worked. Stretching loosens up tight muscles, increases your range of motion, makes your movements freer and easier, increases circulation, and decreases discomfort. When done correctly, stretching feels good. Never stretch to the point of pain or burning sensation. That kind of stretching can cause microscopic tears in muscles and tendons. The resulting scar tissue will make the muscle even tighter and more inflexible. Stretching too fast or too intensely activates a protective mechanism called the stretch reflex. A nerve impulse causes the muscle to contract strongly to brace itself against injury. So the overstretched muscle actually tightens. Fast, intense stretching does more harm that good. Stretch to the point of mild tension, then relax as you hold the stretch. Focus your attention on the muscle being stretched and try to sustain a relaxed stretch for ten to thirty seconds. The feeling of tension should subside as you relax. If it doesn't, ease up a bit.

- Listen to your body. Some days are more stressful and tiring than others, so you won't always be able to work at the same intensity. If you ever feel pain or discomfort in your neck, shoulders, back, hips, or knees, stop. You should feel your muscles work, but you should never feel discomfort in a joint. Stop, gently shake your limbs out, walk around a few minutes, then try again. If you still feel pain in your joint, then stop for the day.

Precautions for Working with a Resistance Band:

- Always warm up first for five to ten minutes. Gently move your arms and legs by walking, riding an exercise bike, or doing another activity.

- Stretch after each exercise to release tension, improve circulation, and increase flexibility in the muscle group that was just worked. Do one of the relaxation movements described at the end of each section after each set.

- Body alignment is extremely important. Keep your rib cage lifted, but not bowed, your shoulders relaxed and squared, and your abdominals tight and pulled in toward your spine. Keep your head over your shoulders. It is really easy to let your head drop forward. Don't let it.

- The exercises can be performed while sitting in a chair or standing, whichever is more comfortable for you.

- There are three ways you can hold a resistance band. First, you can place it between your thumb and index finger and fold all four fingers over the ends. Second, you can wrap the band around your hand once or twice (this position provides a firm hold but can diminish circulation to your hands; be sure to release the band after each set). Or, you can place an end of the band in the palm of each hand and wrap your fingers over it. Choose the position that is most comfortable for you.

- Don't bend your wrists while doing the exercises. Keep your hands straight to the wrists and don't let them be pulled out of alignment.

- You can make the exercises easier by sliding your hands further away from one another on the band. You can make them more difficult by placing your hands closer together. When you begin, test each exercise with your hands far apart on the band. See how it feels, then adjust your hands according to your level of strength.

- You should check with your doctor before doing resistance exercises if you have a history of high blood pressure, shoulder injury, dislocation, or crepitus (grinding, snapping), or carpal tunnel syndrome.

- Use slow, controlled movements. Never hyperextend or lock the joints. Breathe evenly the whole time. Don't hold your breath.

- Make sure your shoulders don't creep up toward your ears. Keep them re-laxed and pressed down.

Now that you've got the basics, you're ready to get going. Better posture awaits!

Chapter 1

Assessing Your Own Posture

Start by taking a good look at the way you usually stand, either by having a friend take a side-view picture or by standing sideways in front of a full-length mirror. Better yet would be to stand in front of three mirrors, like those found in department store dressing rooms–where you can look straight ahead but see yourself from several angles.

❑ Does your head protrude forward?

❑ Is your upper back hunched forward in a rounded curve?

❑ Do your shoulder blades stick out? One more than the other?

❑ Do your shoulders round over and fall forward?

❑ When you let your arms just hang down, what position are your hands in? Are your palms facing the sides of your thighs, or do they point behind you?

❑ Are your hands directly beside your thighs, or do you hold them more towards the front of your thighs?

❑ Are your shoulders tensed and held up closely to your ears?

❑ Is your abdomen protruding forward into a potbelly?

❑ Is your lower back arched or swayed?

❑ Are your knees locked back?

❑ Do your ankles roll in, causing your arches to flatten?

These are all signs of common posture problems.

Now remove your shoes and stand with your back against a wall. Heels should be no more than an inch or two from the wall.

❏ Are there more than a few inches gap between your lower back and the wall?

❏ Do your shoulders touch the wall? Is there more space behind one shoulder than the other?

❏ Can you touch the back of your head to the wall without arching your neck?

❏ Are there more than a few inches space between the back of your neck and the wall?

Any of the above would indicate you have lots to gain by improving your posture.

Don't be discouraged. No matter how bad you think your posture is or how long you've had poor posture, it is never too late. You can improve your posture and you can start right now. In the next chapter, we'll take a look at what good posture/good alignment really looks like.

Chapter 2

What is Good Posture?

Examine your standing posture. Your spine and joints are in alignment when, from a side view:

- Your ear, shoulder, hip, knee, and ankle are in a straight line.

- Your head is directly on top of your shoulders.

- Your upper back is fairly straight (not slouched).

- Your shoulder blades are lying flat against your back.

- Your shoulders are straight and relaxed.

- Your pelvis is in a neutral position, meaning the little bony protrusions toward the top of the pelvic bones line up vertically with your pubic bones. (To learn more, see chapter seven.)

- Your knees are unlocked.

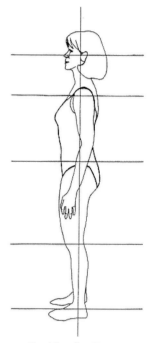

Good Standing Posture

Seated Posture

When you sit you want to maintain the natural curves of your spine. You are sitting correctly when:

- Your ear, shoulder, and hip are in a straight line.
- Your head is centered over your shoulders, not dropped forward.
- Your rib cage is lifted.
- Your arms are supported by armrests.
- Your shoulders are relaxed.
- Your bottom is against the back of the chair.
- Your pelvis is in a neutral position.
- Your thighs are fully supported by the chair seat.
- Your feet are flat on the floor or a stool.

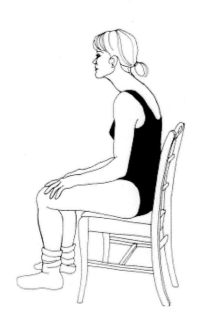

Bad seated posture

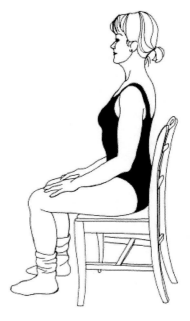

Good seated posture

Now that you know what good posture looks like, how do you get there? You have probably been told many times to sit or stand up straight, but has anyone actually shown you exactly how to achieve this? Chapter three will show you, step-by-step, how to re-align all of your joints so you will be standing straighter instantly. You will see that you can stop the slump, regain lost height, and take an inch or more off your midsection immediately. Let's begin.

Chapter 3

Have Better Posture Instantly

Don't despair if you don't like the way your posture measures up. There's lots you can do to improve your posture right this very minute. Here's how:

One Minute to Better Posture Technique

1. Stand with your feet hip-width apart. Your knees should be soft and neutral, not locked.

2. Pull in your abdominal muscles as if you're zipping up a tight pair of pants. Think of pulling your belly button toward your back. Don't hold your breath.

3. Now you're ready for the most dramatic change. Lift the front of your rib cage up as if there were a string connected from your breastbone to the ceiling, pulling you up. Try to elongate your midsection by pulling the bottom of your rib cage away from your hipbones.

4. Unround your shoulders by externally rotating your arms until your thumbs are in a hitch-hiking position. Gently press your shoulders down, away from your ears. Pull your shoulder blades toward your spine. Then press them down, towards your waist. Next, without letting your shoulders roll forward, relax your arms. Your palms should end up facing your thighs, and your thumbs should end up pointing forward.

5. Finally, gently stretch the top of your head toward the ceiling as if a string were pulling you upward.

6. Keep the position for a few moments, trying to relax into it and breathing normally. Then shake yourself a bit, walk around the room for a few minutes, and go through the steps again. The more you practice this, the more comfortable and natural it will feel.

The One Minute To Better Posture technique will get your ear, shoulder, hip, knee, and ankle in a direct line. It will help you have better posture immediately. If your spinal curves are very accentuated, you will need to practice this as well as do the strengthening exercises for a while before everything lines up perfectly. Every time you do the steps, you will strengthen the muscles of your shoulders, back, and abdomen and teach your body the feel of good posture.

At first, the new position will feel a bit awkward. You're asking your body to behave very differently. But it will not take long to retrain your muscles. If you practice the steps several times a day, in a couple of weeks the position will start to feel natural and really good.

Practice walking or marching in place with good alignment. Keep your rib cage lifted.

For Lasting Change

Now you know what good posture looks like. However, if you've been holding yourself incorrectly for years, your muscles won't be able to keep you aligned properly for very long unless you think about your posture all day long. So the next step in this posture program is to strengthen all the muscles that support good posture. It is your muscles that should be keeping your joints in proper alignment.

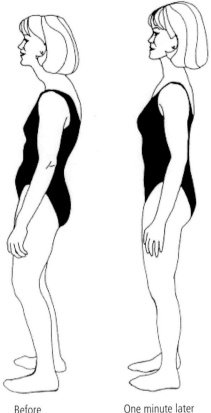

Before   One minute later

> **Instant Alignment Technique**
> When you catch yourself slumping:
> 1. Unlock your knees.
> 2. Pull in your abs.
> 3. Lift your ribcage.
> 4. Unround your shoulders.

The following chapters contain all of the exercises and information needed to beat specific bad posture habits. Each chapter will show you exactly how to align your head over your shoulder or flatten your upper back, un-round and straighten your shoulders, decrease swayback and strengthen your abdominals. Focus on your problem areas. You won't be disappointed.

Part II

Solving Common Posture Problems

Chapter 4

Get Your Head Straight

Have you ever caught your reflection in a window or mirror and noticed your head was leading the way? A head that hangs forward is the most common posture problem. It's caused by many everyday activities, including reading books and newspapers, wearing bifocals, talking on the phone, watching television in bed, working at a computer, and leaning over a desk.

A Real Troublemaker

A head that hangs forward is not only the most widespread posture problem, but also one that causes far more problems than you might think. The reason is that a head is heavy. The average human head weighs ten to fourteen pounds, the same as a bowling ball. It's supposed to rest directly over the shoulders in the body's center of gravity. When it hangs forward even slightly, it is no longer in the center of gravity, and the muscles in the neck and upper back have to work hard all the time just to hold your head up. Every half inch that your head is held in front of your shoulders puts an additional twenty pounds of strain on those muscles. This starts a chain reaction:

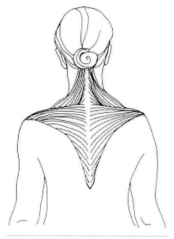

The forward-head position strains the trapezius muscle.

⇨ Most of the work is done by the upper part of the trapezius muscle (trap), a large, diamond-shaped muscle that runs from the base of the skull out to the shoulders and down to the middle back. When the head hangs forward, the upper traps are constantly under tension to hold that heavy load. Over time, they become very thick and tight. When touched, they feel like cement. This causes stiffness and pain in the neck and upper back.

⇨ Because the upper trap is continually contracting, the nerves that pass between the neck bones to serve the arms and upper body get squeezed. The result can be neck pain, numbness or tingling in the arms and hands, or tension headaches. (Tension headaches, the most common type of headache, are often suffered by people whose work requires them to bend or lean forward, such as assembly-line workers, hairdressers, and dentists and dental hygienists.)

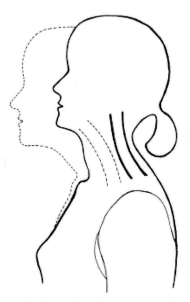

The forward-head position causes the neck to be pulled out of alignment.

⇨ While the upper section of the traps become overdeveloped, the middle and lower parts weaken because they don't have to work at all. The imbalance causes tremendous discomfort in the upper and middle back.

⇨ The splenius cervicus, long, thin muscles that run between the skull and middle back, become stressed and strained and are often felt as hot spots between the shoulder blades.

⇨ When your head hangs forward, unless you want to look at the floor all day, you have to lift your face by arching your neck. This puts pressure on the cartilage, disks, and joints of the neck. Over time, it increases the chance of wear-and-tear arthritis. The constant compression of the disks, nerves, and joints also reduces the flow of blood to the area, cutting down on the oxygen and nutrients that reach the tissues.

> **Everyday Activities that Contribute to Exaggerated Head-Forward Posture**
> Reading Books, Newspapers
> Sewing, Knitting
> Working at a computer
> Crafting, Scrapbooking
> Working at a desk
> Cooking
> Washing dishes
> Driving
> Watching television
> Raking, Shoveling

⇨ The forward-head posture is a major contributor to temporo-mandibular joint disorder (TMJ), which causes pain or clicking noises when you open and close your jaw. TMJ occurs when the hinged joint that connects the lower jawbone to the skull, and the supporting muscles, become inflamed or injured. When the head and jaw are thrust forward, as in the forward-head position, gravity pulls on the jaw and eventually the joint doesn't fit together properly. TMJ can be relieved by realigning the head over the shoulders and relaxing the neck muscles.

⇨ Forward-head posture can lead to tension headaches, neck pain and stiffness, osteoarthritis in the neck, and even bone spurs.

Centering Your Head Over Your Shoulders

Once you're aware of the head-forward problem, it's not difficult to correct. It just takes some attention. Lifting your rib cage, as described in One Minute To Better Posture in chapter three is a great start because it moves your head back closer to your center of gravity. Remember, from a side view your ear and shoulder should be in a straight line. When you re-position your rib cage, you dramatically change what goes on in your neck joints. They fit together the way they are supposed to once again. It will also take immediate tension off your upper back and neck muscles. The following exercises will help re-train your neck muscles and joints. All of the total posture improvement exercises in chapter nine will help you re-align your head over your shoulders. Whenever you think of it throughout the day, gently pull your head back over your shoulders.

Neck Glide

Brings the head back to the center of gravity; greatly relieves neck strain.

1. While standing or sitting, simply pull your head back over the middle of your shoulders. Think of trying to touch an imaginary wall with the back of your neck. Don't tip your head back.

2. Hold position for ten seconds without holding your breath. Do this many times throughout the day.

Putting Your Head in Its Place

Do this whenever you catch yourself with your head hanging forward—for example, when you lean over a desk, computer, or reading material.

1. Sit in a chair, but don't rest against the back. Lift your rib cage up. Pull your belly button toward your spine.

2. Stick your chin forward, then gently pull back your head and neck. Don't tip your head back or arch your neck. Instead, pretend you're trying to touch the back of your neck to an imaginary wall behind you.

3. Keeping your head high, feel the back of your neck gently stretch and your upper back flatten.

4. Push down on your knees with your hands to help your back become as erect as possible. Hold position for five seconds without holding your breath. Relax and repeat several times.

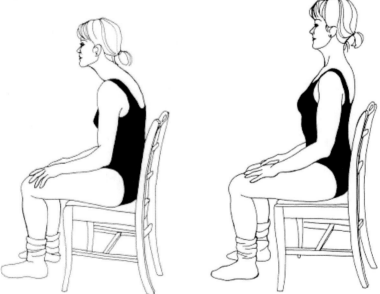

Putting Your Head in Its Place

Neck Glide with Resistance

1. Slide your bottom all the way to the back of the chair seat. Lift your rib cage up. Pull your belly button toward your spine.

2. Place your hands at the back of your head.

3. Gently press the back of your head into your hands using your hands as resistance.

4. Hold position for three to five seconds without holding your breath. Relax and repeat several times.

Neck Stretches

If your head hangs too far forward, you may have extremely tight tendons and muscles in the back and on the sides of your neck, which can be the source of much neck discomfort and of tension headaches. Once you get more flexibility in the neck muscles, you'll be amazed at how much neck discomfort will just fall away.

Stretching exercises will reduce the muscle tension. Do the following stretches gently, adjusting to your level of flexibility. Stretch until you feel mild tension—you should never feel discomfort. Focus your attention on the area being stretched. Try to relax the muscles as you stretch them. Do not yank on your head or neck or you will defeat the purpose of the stretches. Gradually, you will gain flexibility.

Neck Stretch #1: Trapezius Stretch
Stretches the sides of the neck and upper trap muscle.

1. Sit erect in a chair.

2. To stretch the right side of your neck, drop your left ear toward your left shoulder. Press your right shoulder down and reach away slightly with your right arm.

3. Place your left hand over your head and by your right ear. Don't yank on your head with your hand but just feel the weight of your hand adding to the stretch.

4. To finish this off, gently turn your nose towards your left nipple. Hold for ten seconds without holding your breath.

5. Change sides.

6. If you find one side of your neck is much tighter than the other side, stretch the tighter side first and then stretch the other side. Finish by stretching the tighter side again.

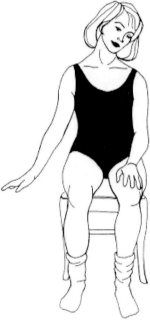

Trapezius Stretch

Neck Stretch #2: Chin-to-Chest Press

Stretches the back and sides of the neck.

1. Sit erect in a chair.

2. To stretch the left side, turn your chin toward your right shoulder. Drop your chin to your chest. Place your right hand on top of your head and gently ease your chin toward your chest (though you won't actually touch your chin to your chest). Don't force this stretch or yank on your head. Even if your chin moves only ¼ inch towards your chest, that's fine for now. The more you do this, the further you'll get. Hold position for ten seconds without holding your breath and release.

3. Repeat on the opposite side.

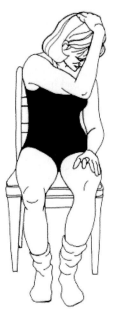

Chin-to-Chest Press

Raking Relaxation Technique

This little massage technique will help relax those really tight, tense neck muscles. Do it between each neck stretch.

1. Place the fingers of both hands at the back of your neck. Right hand fingers should be along the right side of neck muscles and left hand fingers along the left side.

2. Rake your fingers across those muscles. Move from neck bones laterally to the outside of neck.

3. Comfortably dig your fingers into those muscles as you rake.

4. Comfortably rake for ten to fifteen seconds.

Massage Along the Ridge of Your Skull

This massage technique will help relieve tension from some of the spots where muscles insert into the skull. If you feel sore, tender spots along the ridge, this means those muscles are overworked. This massage will help release some of that tension and help work out any inflammation.

1. Along the edge of your skull there is a ridge. Place each index finger on the center of that ridge.

2. Start doing little circular movements with your fingers. Work from the center of the ridge towards your ears. Don't be surprised if you feel some really tender, sore spots along that ridge.

3. Do circular massage back down the ridge towards the center again.

Helpful Hint

To help you practice your head/neck alignment, try this: Whenever you have five or ten minutes, pull your head back over your shoulders, as in the Neck Glide exercise. Have a tape dispenser handy. Pull off a three- to four-inch piece of tape and, with your head held directly over your shoulders, place the piece of tape along the back of your neck. As you go about your business for the next five minutes or so, if you let your head fall forward even a little, you will feel the tape pull, which will alert you to pull your head back over your shoulders. If you can keep your head directly over your shoulders for even five minutes at a time, this will go a long way in re-training the joints and muscles in your neck to do the right thing.

Chapter 5

Stop Slumping

Another very common posture problem is a slumped upper back. Straightening the upper back will decrease waist measurement, increase chest measurement, restore height, provide more space for the lungs and other internal organs, and decrease those annoying, nagging aches and pains that go along with poor posture.

In a Slump

When the upper back slumps forward, it causes a lot of problems.

- The front of the rib cage presses down on the midsection causing the midsection to widen and the belly to protrude. Standing tall eliminates the pressure on the abdominal organs, which instantly slims the waistline. You instantly lose one or more inches around the middle.

- Slumping forward exaggerates the curve in the upper part of your spine. You can *lose as much as two inches in height*, depending on how rounded your upper back is. This happens to many people as they age. If you have lost height over the years, chances are your spinal curves have become too exaggerated. You can regain most of this height by correcting your posture.

- Slumping instantly *decreases your chest measurement.*

- Slumping causes the *shoulders to become rounded and narrow.*

- Slumping forces your head forward of your shoulders. This is the source of much neck pain and discomfort as it causes neck muscles to work *incredibly hard all day long, leaving them tense and stiff.*

- Slumping causes your *clothes to fit poorly.*

- Slumping can decrease breathing capacity by as much as 30 percent. When your chest slumps forward, your rib cage cannot expand as much as it once did, and you become a *shallow breather*. Less oxygen reaches your brain and therefore your body has less energy.

- The downward pressure *gives your heart, liver, and stomach less room, too*.

Exercises to Straighten Up

When the upper back slumps forward, the muscles across the middle back and between the shoulder blades are constantly in a stretched position. They become weak and loose. The muscles in the front of the shoulders and across the chest are always contracted, so they become too short and tight. If your chest slumps forward, you need to strengthen the muscles across the middle back and between your shoulder blades, and stretch the muscles in the front of your chest.

Wall Push-Up

Strengthens the back, chest, and arms. Caution: Skip this exercise if you have carpal tunnel syndrome.

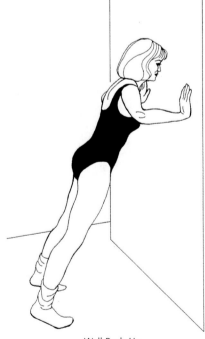

1. Face the wall. Bend your knees slightly and pull in your abdominals so your pelvis is in a neutral position, not tipped forward. To make this exercise more difficult, move your feet farther away from the wall. To make it easier, move your feet closer to the wall.

2. Place your hands against the wall at shoulder level, at a distance apart of a few inches wider than your shoulders. Bend your elbows and lower your torso to the wall. Try to flatten your upper back between the shoulder blades as you lean toward the wall. Don't let your lower back sag.

3. Exhale slowly and push your body away from the wall without letting your elbows lock.

4. Repeat ten times, and gradually build to twenty-five times.

Wall Push-Up

Elbow Press

Strengthens the mid- and upper back muscles.

1. Sit in a chair. Clasp hands behind your head.

2. Lift rib cage up slightly. Relax shoulders and neck muscles.

3. Gently press the back of your head into your hands. Feel the muscles down the length of your spine tighten.

4. Next, press your elbows back, in little pulses, ten times. Your elbows won't move far, but they don't have to.

5. Relax by doing the Rhomboid Release stretch (directions at end of this chapter).

Elbow Press

Mid-back and Shoulder Strengthener

This exercise requires the use of a resistance band.

1. Sit in a chair and slide your bottom to the back of the seat until it touches the chair back. Lift rib cage up and let your shoulders and neck relax.

2. Hold the band across the palms of your hands.

3. Lift your arms out to chest level.

4. Pull your hands away from one another as much as possible.

5. Hold for three seconds. Repeat eight to ten times.

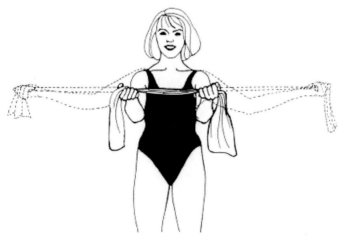

Mid-back and Shoulder Strengthener

Resistance Band Rowing Exercise

This exercise requires the use of a resistance band.

1. Sit in a chair and extend your right leg. Loop your resistance band over your right foot.

2. Lift your rib cage up and let your neck and shoulders relax.

3. Pull your fists straight back toward the sides of your rib cage. Feel the muscles between your shoulder blades contract and tighten as you pull back.

4. Hold the contraction for a slow count of three and relax.

5. Repeat eight to ten times. The slower you do resistance exercises, the more effective they are.

6. Remove band from right foot and loop band over left foot. Lift rib cage, relax shoulders and neck muscles. Lift elbows out from your sides about six inches.

7. Pull your elbows back, feeling the mid-back muscles contract.

8. Release and repeat eight to ten times.

Rhomboid Squeeze

Strengthens the mid-back. This exercise requires the use of a resistance band.

1. Sit in a chair, lift rib cage, and relax shoulders and neck muscles.

2. Grab band and lift elbows from side until they are in a ninety-degree angle with your torso.

3. Pull your elbows back. Squeeze between your shoulder blades as you do this.

4. Repeat eight to ten times.

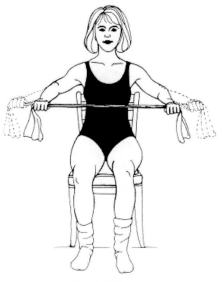

Rhomboid Squeeze

Upper Back Arch

Strengthens muscles between shoulder blades and in the middle back; stretches the chest and the front of the shoulders.

1. Lie on your back with your knees bent and feet flat on the floor. Stretch out your arms at shoulder level with your palms facing up.

2. Gently press all of your spine to the floor, starting with your lower back, then mid-back, upper back, and neck. Keep your chin pulled in and your abdominal muscles tight.

3. Arch the upper back slightly. Try to lift your shoulder blades slightly off the floor. Do not let the lower back or neck arch off the floor. Hold position for a slow count of five without holding your breath. Relax. Repeat two to three times.

Relaxation Stretches

Do one of these between every strengthening exercise in this chapter.

Rhomboid Release

Stretches mid-back muscles.

1. While sitting or standing, interlace your fingers with palms facing out.

2. Stretch arms out in front of your chest. Don't let upper back round forward. Stretch out with your arms and feel the muscles between your shoulder blades stretch.

3. Slide hands to the left and then to the right.

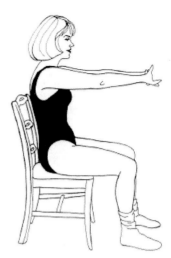

Rhomboid Release

Door Frame Stretch

Stretches tight muscles in the front of the chest and shoulders.

1. Stand in a doorway. Stretch out your arms at shoulder level. Bend your elbows at a ninety-degree angle, so your fingers point toward the ceiling. Place your palms onto the door frame. Tuck your pelvic under by tightening your abdominal muscles.

2. Lean your body forward until you feel a stretch in the front of your shoulders and chest. Hold for ten seconds, then relax.

3. Next, slide your elbows a few inches higher. Lean your torso forward until you feel a stretch in the front of your shoulders. Hold for ten seconds without holding your breath, then relax.

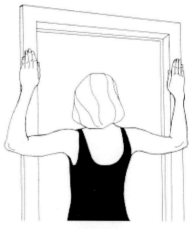

Door Frame Stretch

Deep Breathing Exercise

Deep breathing causes all of the joints along the front and back of your rib cage to move naturally. Helps keep rib and spinal joints mobile and relieves stress and tension not only from the muscles but from your nervous system as well.

1. Inhale through your nose. Think of pulling the oxygen all the way down to the bottom of your rib cage. As you continue to inhale, you should also feel your rib cage expand as your lungs fill with air. See how much you can actually expand your rib cage.

2. Exhale through your mouth. Think of letting all the tension out of neck and back muscles as you exhale. Repeat several times.

3. Next, inhale to a slow count of four and hold your breath for a slow count of four. Exhale for a slow count of four and hold your breath out, gently, for a slow count of four. Repeat several times.

Helpful Hint

Because the rib cage position is hugely important to good posture, here's a tip to help you practice good rib cage alignment and strengthen the muscles that will hold you upright. Whenever you have ten to fifteen minutes at home, lift your rib cage up. Take a string or ribbon and pin it to your shirt just above chest level. Pull the ribbon taut and pin the bottom end just above your waistline. For the next ten or fifteen minutes, just go about your business. Whenever you notice any slack in the ribbon, you will know you are slumping and can reposition. If you can hold your rib cage in the correct position for this amount of time, it will go a long way in strengthening all the muscles that are supposed to hold you upright in the first place.

Chapter 6

Straighten Your Shoulders

Many people round their shoulders forward or carry one higher than the other.

Rounded Shoulders

The shoulder contains not one joint, but several. They all work together whenever you move your arms.

When the shoulders are rounded, the arm bones rotate inward too much. To feel what I'm talking about, place a hand on the opposite shoulder. Rotate your arm externally, until your thumb is pointing out as if you were hitchhiking. As you rotate your arm outward, you should feel the front of your shoulder widen and flatten. You'll feel your shoulder blades retract and lie flatter. Now let the arm bone rotate inward all the

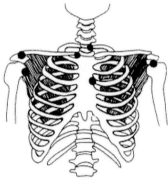

Joints affected by the shoulder

way and feel what that does to your shoulder. The front of the shoulder sort of folds in on itself and the back of the shoulder becomes rounded. When your arms are rotated out slightly, or in a neutral position, your shoulders will feel wider and lie flatter. Your chest is allowed to expand, giving your lungs more room. You'll breathe more deeply.

Rounded shoulders will stretch and weaken the muscles in the back of the shoulders and between the shoulder blades and cause the shoulder blades to be held higher and farther apart than they should be. The inside edges can protrude like wings instead of lying flat. On the front of the body, the shoulder muscles are constantly contracting, so they become too short and too tight.

Many people mistakenly believe the way to straighten up is to jam their shoulders back, like a soldier—but this just causes tension in the neck. To realign all the shoulder joints, you have to rotate the arm outward and gently squeeze your shoulder blades together.

If you want to know whether your shoulders are too rounded, stand and let your arms hang naturally by your sides. Where are your hands? Are they more towards the front of your thighs or directly beside your thighs? Is the front of your hand facing forward with your thumbs touching the thighs? If so, your shoulders are too rounded. The Shoulder Straightener exercise will easily help you realign them.

As you do these exercises, or any in this book for that matter, make sure you keep your head and neck pulled back and centered over your shoulders. If your head is allowed to drop forward, the chest sinks and rounded shoulders become more exaggerated—just what you don't want.

Exercises
Shoulder Straightener
Instantly unrounds the shoulders.

1. Stand with your arms hanging loosely at your sides. Lift your rib cage. Pull your head and neck back until your head is directly over your shoulders.

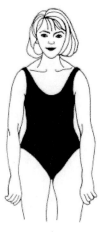
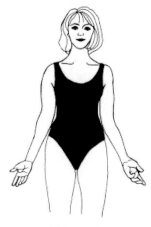
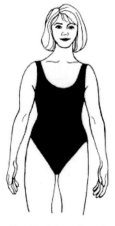

Rounded shoulders Hitchhiker position Shoulder joints aligned

2. Rotate your arms outward. Your thumbs should be pointing out as if you were hitchhiking.

3. Press both shoulders down, away from your ears.

4. Without letting your shoulders roll forward, let your arms relax. Your arm bones will roll in to a neutral position. Your palms should face your thighs, and your thumbs should be pointing straight ahead. This is the anatomically correct position of the arms and hands when the shoulders are correctly aligned. If the thumbs are pointing ahead, and if your chest feels expanded and your shoulders wider, you've done it right.

While the Shoulder Straightener instantly unrounds the shoulders, as soon as you start thinking about something else, your shoulders will go back to their old ways. So the next step is to strengthen the muscles in the back of your shoulders and between your shoulder blades and stretch the muscles in the front of your shoulders. The goal is to obtain a balance so your muscles can hold your shoulders in place without you giving them a thought.

The Hitchhiker

Strengthens the large muscles across the upper and mid-back and helps unround the shoulders.

1. Sit on a chair. Grab the chair seat and pull your chest up and slightly forward. Bring your head over your shoulders. Elongate your midsection. Inhale deeply. As you exhale, keep your rib cage lifted, and tighten your abdominals.

2. Breathing normally, rotate your arms until your thumbs point behind you. Hunch your shoulders up towards your ears and then press them down.

3. Press your arms back in little movements from one to twenty times. Think of squeezing your shoulder blades toward one another each time.

4. Relax by letting your torso lean forward on your legs. Let your arms hang like deadweights.

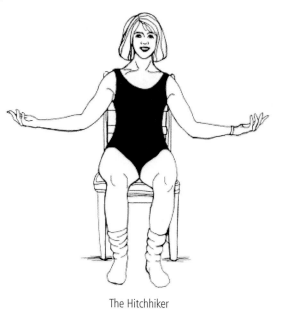

The Hitchhiker

Elbow Press

Strengthens muscles in mid- and upper back as well as back of shoulders.

1. Sit on a chair.

2. Clasp your hands behind your head. Lift your shoulders toward your ears and then press them down away from your ears. (If you feel the muscles in the back of your neck tighten while doing the rest of this exercise, you are holding your shoulders too high. Relax them and press them down. If the problem continues, skip this exercise for now and do the Hitchhiker exercise for a few weeks instead.)

3. Gently press the back of your head into your hands. You should feel the muscles along your spine tighten. Hold position for five seconds without holding your breath.

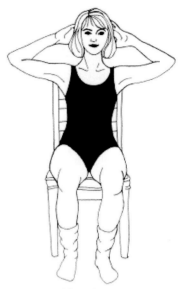

Elbow Press

4. Next, press your elbows back ten times. They won't move very far, but you'll feel this in the muscles between your shoulder blades.

5. Relax by letting your torso lean forward and rest on your thighs. Repeat several times.

Rotator Cuff Strengthener

This exercise requires the use of a resistance band. Strengthens rotator cuff muscles.

1. Lift your rib cage up, press your shoulders away from your ears, and tighten your abdominals. Elbows should be by your sides, with forearms in a ninety-degree angle to upper arm.

2. With palms facing up, let band lie across your palms. Tighten fingers around band.

3. Keeping elbows close to your sides, pull hands away from one another. Hold position for a slow count of three but don't hold your breath.

4. Release and repeat eight to ten times.

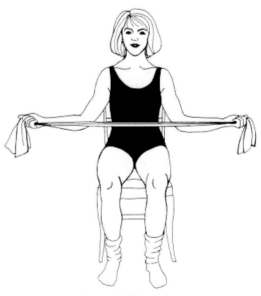

Rotator Cuff Strengthener

Bow and Arrow

This exercise requires the use of a resistance band. Strengthens shoulders and mid- and upper back.

1. Lift your rib cage up and align your head over your shoulders. Press your shoulders down and tighten your abs.

2. Grab the band with your left hand and extend that arm in front of your body slightly above chest level, keeping the elbows slightly bent.

3. Grab the other end of the band with your right hand. Pull your right elbow back and down in one smooth motion. Hold position for a few seconds without holding your breath. Release and repeat eight to ten times.

4. Change arms and repeat steps one through three.

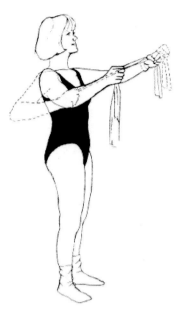

Bow and Arrow

Shoulder Raises

This exercise requires the use of a resistance band. Strengthens shoulders and corrects rounded shoulders.

1. Stand with your feet hip-width apart, knees slightly bent, abdominals pulled in, rib cage lifted, head aligned.

2. With your arms hanging by your sides, grab the band with your hands. Gently pull your shoulder blades towards each other and then press them down, away from ears.

3. Holding the band steady with your right hand, raise your left arm without letting your shoulder blades or torso move. Your thumb should point towards the ceiling. At first, raise your arm about forty-five degrees. Hold position for a count of three without holding your breath, then slowly release. As you become stronger, you can raise your arm to just below shoulder level.

4. Repeat eight to ten times.

5. Change arms and repeat steps one through four.

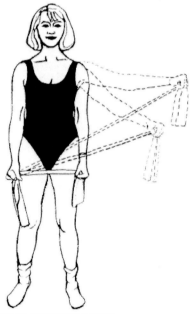

Shoulder Raises

Tricep Strengthener

This exercise requires the use of a resistance band. Strengthens the shoulders and the backs of the arms.

1. Grip the band with your right hand and place that hand on your chest.

2. With the left hand, grab the band six inches away from the other hand.

3. Raise your left elbow a few inches below shoulder level.

4. Extend your forearm until the whole arm is straight. Don't let your shoulders creep up. Keep them pressed down.

5. Hold the position for three seconds without holding your breath, and slowly release.

6. Do eight to ten repetitions.

7. Change arms and repeat steps one through six.

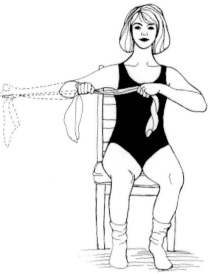

Tricep Strengthener

Stretches

Door Frame Stretch

Stretches the front of the shoulders and the chest.

1. Stand in a doorway. Stretch out your arms at shoulder level. Bend your elbows at a ninety-degree angle, so your fingers point toward the ceiling. Place your palms on the door frame. Tuck your pelvis under by tightening your abdominal muscles.

2. Lean your body forward until you feel a stretch in the front of your shoulders and chest. Hold position for ten seconds without holding your breath, then relax.

3. Next, slide your elbows several inches higher. Lean your torso forward until you feel a stretch in the front of your shoulders. Hold position for ten seconds without holding your breath, then relax.

4. Repeat several times throughout your day.

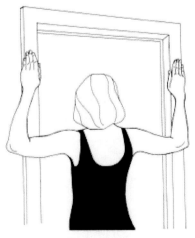

Door Frame Stretch

Chest and Shoulder Stretch

Stretches the front of the shoulders and the chest.

1. Stand erect. Place your hands behind your back, one on top of the other, palms facing up.

2. Press your shoulders down, away from your ears. Lift your arms as far as is comfortable. Hold position for ten seconds without holding your breath, then relax.

Uneven Shoulders

Another common shoulder problem is holding one side higher than the other. Look into a mirror to see if your shoulders are uneven. Uneven shoulders cause a lot of muscle tension. On the side that is higher, the neck muscles are tight and thick, and the muscles of the trunk are stretched. On the other side of the body, the trunk muscles shorten and contract. This muscular imbalance is the source of many back, neck, and shoulder problems.

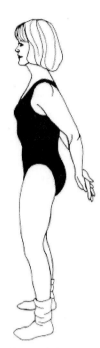

Chest and Shoulder Stretch

To retrain your muscles, simply spend as much time as possible with your shoulders even. Here's an easy way to keep track of your shoulders throughout the day. You'll need a large mirror and some tape. Look in the mirror to see if one shoulder is higher than the other. Pull the higher shoulder down until you can see in the mirror that your shoulders are even. On the side of the once-higher shoulder, put an inconspicuous piece of tape on the place where your fingertips rest on the side of your leg or clothes. Throughout the day, as often as you think of it, let your fingertips find the tape on your leg or clothing. Whenever your fingertips are brushing against the tape, you'll know that your shoulders are even. To check your shoulders while you're sitting, you can pull your shoulders even and place a marker where your elbow rests against your rib cage.

> **Signs of Scoliosis**
>
> Uneven shoulders and uneven hips can be a sign of scoliosis, a medical condition in which the spine is curved sideways. The condition is often present at birth and becomes obvious during childhood or the teen years. If you suspect that you or your child may have scoliosis, see your doctor. Your doctor will refer you to a physical therapist who will evaluate your condition and teach you exercises for your special needs. You may also be referred to an orthopedic surgeon, a doctor who specializes in treating disorders of bones and joints. Don't do the exercises suggested here, and don't ignore the problem. Without treatment, the problem will grow worse, causing back pain and lung problems.

The more time you spend with your shoulders correctly aligned, the more quickly your muscles will be retrained. The tape trick will help you regain your sense of balance, too. At first you'll feel off-balance since you're used to having your shoulders slanted. Soon your body, especially your spine and neck, will come to appreciate correctly aligned shoulders and you won't need the tape as a reminder. In just a few weeks you should see and feel results.

You also need to change habits that probably caused the problem in the first place. Try the following.

- *If you carry a purse, lighten it up, and alternate the shoulder on which you carry it.* The number one cause of uneven shoulders in women is carrying a heavy purse on the same shoulder. To keep the strap from sliding off the shoulder, especially if a woman is round-shouldered, she has to hike up the shoulder. Day after day, year after year, this creates muscular imbalances. The muscles of the higher shoulder become tight and thick, and after a while automatically hold the shoulder in a higher position. Do you really need all that muscle tension?

> **Those Earrings Are Definitely Not You**
> Are you wearing your shoulders like earrings? Asking yourself this question several times a day will help you remember to press your shoulders down and away from ears.

- *Same goes for your briefcase or books.* If you always carry a heavy briefcase or laptop computer on one side, you'll cause stress, strain, and imbalances in the spine. At the very least, switch sides often. To carry books or notebooks to school or around campus, use a backpack instead of a bag.

- *Stand with your weight evenly on both legs.* Many people create uneven shoulders and hips because they always stand with their weight on the same leg. Try to distribute your weight evenly. If you have trouble breaking this habit, at least switch sides—shift your weight to the other leg.

- *Avoid carrying a child on your hip.* This automatically raises the hip and the shoulder on that side. Being a mother, I know the hip position is practical because it leaves a hand free to do things, but I urge you to use it as little as possible. Carry your child in front, close to you, with both arms. If you need to park a kid on your hip sometimes, change hips often. If you find yourself constantly carrying a baby around the house, try a baby backpack, which puts the weight in your center of gravity rather than on one side.

Helpful Hint

To help you practice good shoulder alignment, try this: Whenever you think of it—hopefully many times throughout your day—lift your rib cage. Think of pulling up with your midsection. Pull your shoulder blades back, towards one another and then press them down slightly towards your waistline. You should feel all the muscles between your shoulder blades and in your mid-back contract and tighten. Hold this position for a slow count of ten without holding your breath, then relax. This simple repositioning movement will help strengthen the muscles that, when strong, keep your shoulders in good alignment.

Chapter 7

Lower Back Alignment And Abdominal Strength

Many people experience dull, aching, or shooting pain in the lower back. Back pain can make it difficult to walk, sit, sleep, work—in fact, to do almost anything. It can make life miserable, and can even be disabling.

The number one cause of lower-back pain is not overdoing it (with a sport, workout, or household chore), but rather poor standing or sitting posture. Standing with your knees locked back causes an exaggerated curve in the lower back, often called a swayback. A swayback is enhanced by weak or inflexible muscles in the abdomen, legs, buttocks, and back. You can strengthen or stretch these important muscles so they will support the lower back and hold the pelvis in neutral position.

Poor sitting posture causes the opposite problem. A common mistake people make when they sit is to let their lower back bow or round out behind them. This puts pressure on the front of the spinal disks, causing the jelly-like centers to be forced to the back side. Sitting this way can cause or worsen a herniated disk.

Back Pain Statistics

1. Thirty-one million Americans have low back pain at any given time.
2. Ninety percent of back problems are due to poor posture. It is the number one cause.
3. Back pain is the second most common cause of work days missed due to illness.
4. Back pain is the most common disability in the U.S.
5. The cost that back pain has is estimated to be a staggering fifty billion dollars yearly.

—From the National Institute of Health

If you have intense or chronic pain in your lower back, see your doctor before doing exercise to rule out any serious conditions such as a herniated disk, scoliosis, broken bone, or osteoporosis.

The Anatomy of Your Back

The spine consists of twenty-four interlocking bones called vertebrae. Stacked one upon another, these small bones support the weight of the body. Each vertebra contains four little joints with pain-sensitive linings. Between the vertebrae are circular pads, called disks, composed of a soft jelly enclosed in a tough, fibrous shell. The disks separate the bones and cushion the impact of walking, running, and moving. They're the spine's shock absorbers. In a healthy back, the disks are plump and thick.

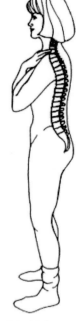

Spinal Column

Inside this column of bones is the spinal cord, a thick bundle of nerves. Smaller nerves pass between the vertebrae and branch out to the rest of the body.

The spine has three slight curves, in the neck (the cervical curve), upper back (thoracic curve), and lower back (lumbar curve). These curves absorb shock and give the spine flexibility, while keeping the column balanced over the center of gravity. When the spine curves just the right amount, the vertebrae are stacked up properly. They glide against each other without friction. When the curves are too great, however, the spinal joints no longer fit together properly and thus press into one another. The joint linings can become irritated and inflamed. Also, because the space between the vertebrae is narrowed when the lower back is swayed, the nerves that pass between them don't have enough room. They're pressed upon and pinched.

Too much curve in the lumbar area causes lower-back pain. If there is compression of the sciatic nerve, the person can feel anything from a dull ache to a stabbing, burning pain in the lower back, buttocks, down the leg, and even into the big toe. There can be a spot or area of pain or a line of pain down the entire leg.

Does Your Lower Back Curve Too Much?

Take this test.

- First, stand with your back and heels against a wall. Is there a tunnel between your lower back and the wall? Can you fit the palm of one hand there? Is there lots of extra room?

- Now look at yourself sideways in a mirror. Does your belly protrude? Your bottom?

- Do your knees lock back?

- Does your back ache after you've been on your feet for a while, for example after you've been to the mall or at a museum?

If you answered yes to any of the above questions, then your lower back curve is probably too exaggerated.

Get Your Pelvis in Neutral

The first step in lessening the curve in your lower back is to get your pelvis in a neutral position. The little bony protrusions toward the top of your pelvic bones (called the iliac crests) should be lined up vertically with your pubic bones when you are standing or sitting, and line up horizontally when you are lying down. Training your pelvis to be in neutral is a big step toward improving your posture and freeing yourself of lower-back discomforts.

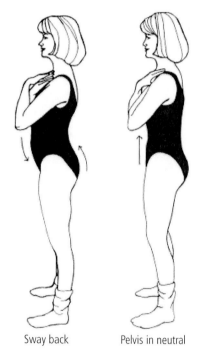

Sway back   Pelvis in neutral

Pelvic tilts are a great place to start. The beginner version is done in the reclining position. When you lie down, gravity assists you, making it easier to lessen the curve in your lower back. In the intermediate version, the wall helps out. If your lower-back curve has been too extreme, the soft tissue and muscles in the small of your back may have become very tight and inflexible. It'll take time to change this. If you feel discomfort while doing the pelvic tilt, stop. Try again, more gently, in a few hours.

Soon you'll be able to do a pelvic tilt without the support of the floor or wall. During the day, whenever you think of it, you'll be able to bring your pelvis into a neutral position, lessening your lower-back curve and taking the pressure off your joints, soft tissues, and nerves. Finally, you'll be able to do an advanced standing pelvic tilt. By not using your buttocks to help tilt your pelvis, you will help your abdominals work harder and become stronger.

Exercises

Pelvic Tilt for Beginners
Strengthens abdominals and takes pressure off lower back joints.

1. Lie on a bed or thick rug. Bend your knees and place your feet flat on the floor. Inhale.

2. As you exhale, squeeze your buttock muscles and tighten your abdominal muscles by pulling your belly button toward your back. Gently press your lower back into the floor until the pelvic and pubic bones line up horizontally.

3. Hold your muscles tight for a count of ten without holding your breath, and release. Repeat several times.

Pelvic Tilt, Intermediate Level

1. Stand with your back against a wall. Place your heels about six inches from the wall and bend your knees slightly.

2. Pull your belly button toward your spine and gently, slowly coax your lower back against the wall. Don't force anything. At first, you may have to bend your knees a lot and place your heels far away from the wall (up to twelve inches). With time, you'll be able to bend your knees less and get your feet closer to the wall.

3. Hold position for ten seconds without holding your breath. Relax.

Advanced Standing Pelvic Tilt

1. Stand with your feet hip-width apart and your knees unlocked.

2. Pull your belly button toward your back and tighten your abdominal muscles.

3. Drop your tailbone slightly. This eases the pelvis into a neutral position.

Tilt Tip

How can you know whether you're doing a standing pelvic tilt properly? Place your hands on your abdomen. Put your thumbs on the bottom of your rib cage, and your other fingers on your hipbones. As you tilt your pelvis, your fingers and thumbs should move closer together.

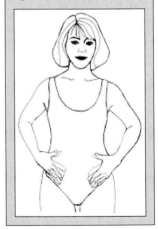

4. Hold for a slow count of five, then relax. As you become more experienced, increase the count to thirty, then for as long as you can. Try to relax your buttocks while keeping your abs tight and your hips tucked under. Don't hold your breath. Let all the other muscles in your body relax while still keeping the abdominals tight.

5. Hold for ten seconds without holding your breath. Relax and repeat several times.

The next step is to train your oblique muscles, the stabilizers, to keep your pelvis in neutral while your other body parts are moving and going about their daily business. When strong, these muscles that wrap around the sides of the body keep your pelvis balanced and stable. They provide tremendous support for the lower back.

The following exercises will help strengthen your oblique muscles. If the exercises feel easy, you're probably allowing your pelvis to move rather than keeping it perfectly still and in neutral. Have someone check you as you move your legs. The slower you exercise, the more effective you'll be, and the better you'll be able to keep your pelvis in neutral.

Ab Stabilizer, Level 1
Strengthens the oblique muscles.

1. Lie on your back, knees bent, feet flat on the floor, arms by your sides.

2. Make sure your pelvis is in neutral, then tighten your abs. Keeping the abs tight and without moving your pelvis, slowly pull one knee toward your chest. Tighten the abs even more, then place that foot back on the floor without letting the pelvis move. If it moves even a little, the purpose of the exercise is defeated.

3. Switch knees. Do five sets. Try not to hold your breath at any point during the exercise.

Ab Stabilizer, Level 2

1. In the same position as above, without letting the pelvis move, first pull up one knee, then add the other.

2. Again without letting the pelvis move even slightly, place the right foot back on the floor, then the left foot. To accomplish this, you must hold your abs in extremely tight.

3. Do five sets. Try not to hold your breath at any point during the exercise.

Ab Stabilizer, Level 3

1. Start in the same position. Keeping the knee bent at a ninety-degree angle, lift your right leg until the calf is parallel to the floor. At the same time, exhale and raise your left arm over your head. Do not let your pelvis move even a little.

2. Inhaling, bring the arm and leg back to the starting position.

3. Repeat with the opposite arm and leg.

4. See if you can do both sides three times. Gradually, build to eight times.

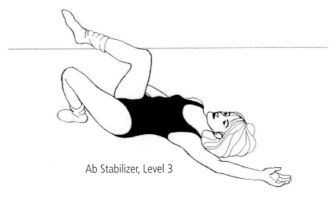

Ab Stabilizer, Level 3

Standing Stabilizer

Trains the oblique muscles to keep the pelvis in neutral.

1. Stand against a wall with your pelvis in neutral and rib cage lifted.

2. Lift your arms in front of you. Without letting your pelvis or lower back move from the wall, lift your arms overhead. Lift only as far as you can and still keep your pelvis in neutral. At first, you may be surprised to find that you can't lift very far without your lower back coming away from the wall. Keep practicing. As your oblique muscles grow stronger, you'll be able to lift your arms higher while still keeping your pelvis neutral.

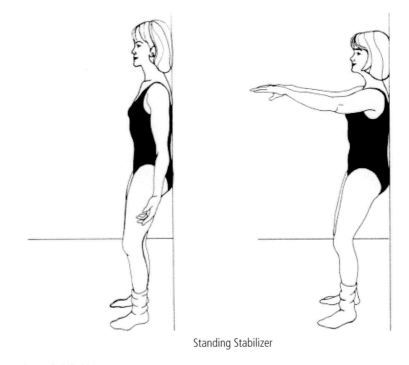

Standing Stabilizer

Stretches

Tight, shortened muscles in the lower back lock the pelvis into a forward tilt. The exercises described below will help relax the lower back and stretch lower-back muscles. Do them whenever you can. They feel great if you've been on your feet for a while or if you've been standing on concrete floors.

Rock and Roll

Stretches the lower back; this feels really good, since it relieves pressure in the spinal joints and soft tissues.

1. Lie on your back and bend your knees towards your abdomen.

2. Place your hands behind your knees in towards your chest.

3. Gently rock your knees towards your chest for a few seconds.

4. Gently ease your knees towards your chest as far as they'll comfortably go.
   Hold for ten to twenty seconds and feel your lower back stretch. Don't hold your breath.

Rock and Roll

5. Next, guide your knees in a circle over your chest five times in one direction and five times in the other direction.

Sink Stretch

Stretches the whole spine and feels great.

1. Hold on to the rim of a sink with your feet directly under your shoulders, hip-width apart. Tuck your hips under and bend your knees a bit.

2. Let your bottom sink back slightly as if you were about to sit on the floor. Your arms should straighten but not lock. Relax your neck muscles so your head hangs down a bit and you feel a stretch down your spine. Hold this position for ten seconds as you let your back relax. Do not hold your breath.

3. Ease back to a standing position. Repeat several times throughout the day.

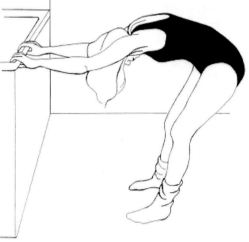

Sink Stretch

Exercises

There are four layers of abdominal muscles, each with fibers running in different directions. The crisscrossing pattern shapes your midsection and supports your lower back. When the abdominal muscles are weak, the lower back sags inward, which puts uneven pressure on the joints in the small of your back and causes your belly to stick out more.

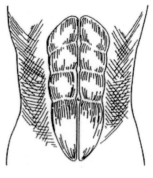

Abdominals

Strong abdominals contribute greatly to the health of the total spine. The Pelvic Tilts and Ab Stablizers will help. Also, do any of the Abdominal Strengtheners often throughout the day. They will help you strengthen all four layers of abdominal muscle.

Abdominal Strengthener #1

Strengthens the abdominal muscles to keep your lower back safe and pain-free. It even strengthens the deepest layer, called the Transverse Abdominus. Crunches don't even touch this layer. This exercise is totally inconspicuous and should be done as often throughout the day as you think of it.

1. Take in a deep breath. Feel your rib cage expand as your lungs fill with air.

2. As you exhale through your mouth, pull your abdominals in as if you were trying to zip up a really tight pair of pants. Pull your belly button toward your spine and feel the bottom edge of your rib cage pull in and decrease in diameter. Hold your abdominals as tightly as you can while you slowly count to five, then relax. Gradually build up to twenty seconds. Practice holding your abdominals in tightly while still taking breaths. Don't hold your breath.

Abdominal Strengthener #2

1. Inhale through your nose. Think of pulling the oxygen all the way down to the bottom of your rib cage. As you continue to inhale, you should feel your rib cage expand.

2. Exhale through your mouth, like you were pushing air through a straw. As you exhale, pull your belly button towards your spine.

3. Try to push a little more air out—then a little more—and then a little more. As you gently force the air out of your rib cage, you will feel all the abdominal muscles as well as the bottom of your rib cage pull in.

4. Hold the abdominals in tightly for a slow count of ten without holding your breath. Then relax and repeat several times.

Abdominal Strengthener #3

1. Sit in a chair, lift your rib cage, and press your shoulders down.

2. Place both hands on your left knee.

3. Inhale. As you exhale, begin to pull abdominals in. At the same time, try to lift your left knee but resist the movement with your hands. It will be a bit like a struggle between your knee and your hands.

4. As you lift the knee, resist with your hands and pull your abdominals in as tightly as possible. Hold for a slow count of three without holding your breath. Relax.

5. Place both hands on your right knee and repeat steps one through four.

Abdominal Strengthener #4

1. Sit in a chair, lift your rib cage, and press your shoulders down.

2. Place both hands on the inside of your left knee.

3. Inhale. As you exhale, begin to pull your abdominals in. At the same time, try to drag your left knee towards the right knee but resist with your hands. Hold for a slow count of three without holding your breath.

4. Place both hands on the inside of your right knee and repeat.

How to Do a Proper Crunch

Many people stop doing crunches, not because their abs get tired, but because their neck feels uncomfortable. The way crunches are typically done, the head is pulled forward and the shoulders and upper back are forced into a rounded position. Essentially, they're exercising in really poor alignment, which only makes their posture problems worse.

Please note that the slower you do abdominal exercises, the more effective they are. If you are doing crunches quickly, to the beat of the music, you are wasting your time.

1. Place an apple or a tennis ball under your chin. This will keep your head aligned with your shoulders as you lift up.

2. Clasp your hands behind your head and press your elbows back. Make sure your elbows are pressed back far enough so you cannot see them with your peripheral vision. If at any time during the crunch you can see your elbows, that means you are rounding your shoulders and trying to use your arms to lift your torso. You don't want to do this. Keep your elbows pressed back and try not to use your arms to lift you up.

3. Tighten abs by pulling your belly button towards your spine.

4. Lift your head and shoulders off the floor. As you lift, pull your belly button towards your spine. Hold at the top of the contraction for a slow count of three.

5. Come most of the way down, then repeat eight to ten times. Exhale as you lift up and inhale as you roll back down.

Strengthen Your Buttock Muscles

The buttock muscles (gluteus maximus, medius, and mininus) also help keep the pelvic in a neutral position. When the buttock muscles are weak, they allow the pelvis to tip forward, accentuating the curve of the lower back. Again, the Pelvic Tilts will help. Also do the Buttock Clencher. It takes only a few seconds and can be done many times throughout the day. People who sit for many hours each day (including office workers) usually have weak, flabby butt muscles. This exercise will help counteract the harmful effects of sitting for hours every day.

Buttock Clencher
Strengthens the abdominal muscles, stretches the lower back, and strengthens the buttocks.

1. Stand with your feet hip-width apart, knees slightly bent. Inhale.

2. As you exhale, pull your abdominals in and clench your buttock muscles. This brings your pelvis into a neutral position and lessens the curve in your lower back.

3. Hold for a slow count of ten without holding your breath, then release.

4. Repeat as many times as you can throughout the day.

Unlock Your Knees

Yet another cause of swayback is locking the knees. When a person stands with locked knees, the head of the thighbone (femur) rests against the back of the hip socket, tilting the pelvis forward and arching the lower back. Your knees are locked back if you stand with all of your weight on your heels. This position can also cause knee problems because your kneecaps are smashed back into your leg bones. Whenever you catch yourself standing with your knees locked back, adjust your weight so it is spread evenly over your feet. You don't have to stand with your knees bent, but they should be in a relaxed position, not stiff and pressed backward. For more about the knees, see chapter eight.

Muscles That Can Pull the Pelvis out of Alignment

The quadriceps, hamstrings, and hip flexors are three muscle groups that, when too tight, can pull your pelvis out of neutral.

The quadriceps (quads) are four muscles on the front and sides of the thigh. If the quads are very tight, they limit the range of motion in the hip joint. To accommodate the hips' decreased range of motion, the lower back has to arch and move with every step. This puts a lot of stress and strain on the lower back.

The hamstrings are muscles that go from the back of the lower pelvic bone to just below the back of the knee. When you take a step, they extend the thighs and bend the knees. Tight hamstrings also restrict the range of motion of the hip socket and pull on the lower back. The lower back takes the stress and strain with each step you take. To see whether your hamstrings are tight, lie on your back with your right leg bent and right foot on the floor. Extend your left leg along the floor. Keeping your left leg straight, raise it and see how far it goes while still straight. The goal is to be able to bring your leg to a ninety-degree angle while keeping the knee straight and the foot flexed. Most people have to build up to this because their hamstrings are too tight. Below is a description of the Hamstring Stretch, a simple exercise that can be done at the beginning and end of the day to gain flexibility quickly. You can read something while you are doing it, so your mind is not on your hamstrings and the muscles will be allowed to relax as they stretch. You'll notice an improvement in the comfort of your lower back when your hamstrings are no longer too tight.

The hip flexors (iliopsoas muscles) allow you to raise a bent knee toward your chest. They are large muscles that run from the lower spine, through the abdominal cavity, to the inside of your upper thigh. When they are too tight, they pull your lower back into an arch. Tight hip flexors are very common. Ironically, athletic activity is often a contributing factor.

Stretches

Reclining Quad and Flexor Stretch

Stretches the quadriceps and hip flexors.

1. Lie on your right side and rest the side of your head in the palm of your hand or on your right arm, whichever is more comfortable.

2. Bend your left leg and grab your left ankle with your left hand. Ease the left thigh back as far as is comfortable. Keep the left thigh parallel to the floor.

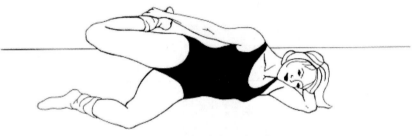

Reclining Quad and Flexor Stretch

3. Hold for ten seconds without holding your breath and release.

4. Change sides and repeat steps one through three.

Standing Quad and Flexor Stretch

Stretches the quadriceps and hip flexors.

1. Place your left hand on a wall or a chair back for balance. Bend your right knee and raise your foot behind you. Grab your right ankle with your right hand and ease your right foot as close to your buttocks as is comfortable. Your knees should be side by side, and your trunk vertical (not leaning forward or back). Make sure the standing leg is slightly bent, not locked. You'll feel a stretch up the front of your leg and in the front of your hip. To increase the stretch, press your hips forward slightly.

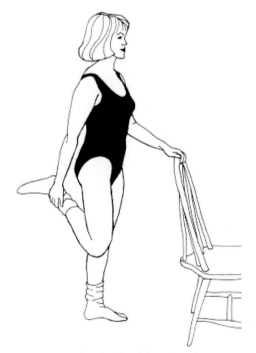

Standing Quad and Flexor Stretch

2. Hold for ten seconds without holding your breath. Over time, build up to twenty seconds. Release and change legs.

3. Repeat steps one and two.

4. If one leg is tighter than the other, spend more time on it.

Hamstring Stretch

Increases flexibility in the hamstrings.

1. Grab a book or magazine before you start. Place a thick rug or mat by a doorway.

2. Lie on your back with your bottom about twelve inches away from the doorjamb. Put one leg through the opening of the door. Bend that leg, and put the foot flat on the floor. Place the other leg up the side of the door. Adjust your position closer to the wall or farther away until you feel a good, comfortable stretch down the back of the raised leg. If you feel this more behind your knee than anywhere else, the stretch is too intense and you should slide your bottom farther from the wall. As you become more flexible, bring your buttocks closer and closer to the wall. Soon you'll be able to get your bottom right against the wall with your leg straight up.

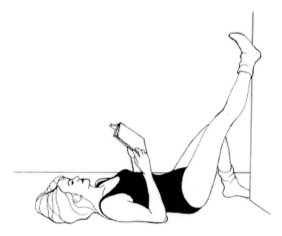

Hamstring Stretch

3. Maintain this position while you read for a minute. If you find your foot begins to tingle, bring that leg down from the wall.

4. Switch legs and repeat.

5. Many people find one leg is tighter than the other. Stretch the tighter leg twice.

Helpful Hint

To help you practice lower back alignment, try this: Whenever you get a spare moment, stand with your back against a wall. Your heels should be about six inches away from the wall and knees slightly bent. Inhale. As you exhale, gently press the small of your back to the wall. To do this, you'll have to tighten your abdominals. Hold this position for ten seconds without holding your breath. To take it a step further, with your lower back pressed gently towards the wall, begin to lift your arms in front of you. As your arms come up, your lower back will want to come away from the wall. Don't let it. At first, you may be surprised to find that you can't lift very far without your lower back coming away from the wall. Keep practicing. As your internal and external oblique muscles grow stronger, you'll be ale to lift your arms higher while still keeping your pelvic in neutral.

Chapter 8

Your Knees, Feet, and Ankles

Correct alignment begins at your base; that is, your knees, ankles, and feet. They have to support the weight of your entire body. If they aren't aligned properly, all of your other joints have to accommodate and are also thrown out of alignment.

If you have painful knees, ankles, or feet because of an injury or surgery, ask your doctor to refer you to a physical therapist to evaluate your problem and prescribe specific exercises.

Your Knees

Have you taken a good look at your knees lately? Take off your shoes and socks and roll up your pants, then turn sideways and look in a mirror. First, are your knees stiff and locked back? When you stand, your knees should be in an easy, neutral position–not bent or locked back. When your knees are locked back, your weight is basically on your heels and the kneecaps get pressed back into the leg bones. This contributes to a swayback by forcing an arch in the lower back. It weakens the quadriceps because in this position, they don't have to work as much. The abs weaken because they are constantly held in a stretched position. Every time you catch yourself with your knees locked back, release them to an easy position.

Look in the mirror again. Do your kneecaps turn inward toward each other? Do they pull to the outside of the leg? When your knees are aligned properly, the kneecaps point straight ahead. If the kneecaps roll in toward one another, you probably need to strengthen the outside of your thighs and stretch the inside muscles. If the kneecaps pull to the outside of the leg, then the outside of your thighs may be too tight. You need to stretch the outside of your thigh and strengthen the inside.

Bend your knees simultaneously and look down between them. Do they track directly over your feet or do they come to the inside? You should see the big toes of each foot when you look down in this position. If you can't, then the knees are misaligned and every time you bend your knees you are wearing away the joint linings, little by little. Do the following simple movement whenever you have a few spare moments.

Knee Straightener
Realigns knees to ankles.

1. Stand with your feet hip-width apart. Make sure your feet are pointing straight ahead.
2. Press your big toes into the floor.
3. Place your hands on the insides of your thighs.
4. Slowly bend your knees while gently pressing your thighs out with your hands, so the knees go directly over the feet. Keep the big toes pressed into the floor as you do this.
5. Bend and straighten your knees ten to twenty times. Note: If this feels uncomfortable, don't bend as far. If it is still uncomfortable, you need to see a physical therapist.

Quadricep Strengthener
Strengthens the quadriceps without stressing the knee joint.

1. Sit in a chair and slide your bottom all the way to the back of the chair seat. Lift your rib cage up, press your shoulders down, and tighten your abs slightly.
2. Extend your right leg straight out in front of you. Toes should be pointing towards the ceiling.
3. Lift your right thigh off the chair seat eight to ten times.
4. Change legs and repeat steps one through three.

Your Feet

The foot contains twenty-six bones and numerous muscles. Take off your socks and shoes and look at your ankles. Do they roll in? Are your arches flat? Do you have bunions or calluses? Are your toes straight or bent? Does the big toe pull inward toward the other toes? These problems are all related to posture.

Most foot problems are caused by wearing shoes with heels that are too high and toe boxes that are too narrow. Wearing high heels alters the position of every weight-bearing joint in your body. Heels higher than one inch increase a swayback, which leads to lower-back discomfort. The foot slides to the front of the shoe, which puts way too much pressure on the ball of the foot and all the toes. High heels shorten the Achilles tendon on the back of the calf and foot and stretch and weaken the muscles on the front of the ankle, which can lead to shin splints. Heels on shoes also get in the way of your natural stride, which is to place the heel down first, then roll through the ball of the foot.

The lower the heel, the better. Even a one-inch heel causes a twelve-degree tilt in the ankle joint, which, in turn, causes all the other joints to adjust so you don't topple over. If a building were tilted twelve degrees, the doors and windows wouldn't work properly. Of course, a building can't make adjustments as a human body can. Our bodies adjust, but we eventually pay for it with stiff, aching joints and painful feet. The heel of your foot should be as close to the ground as possible.

Wearing footwear with narrow or pointed toe boxes squeezes all of your toes together. When the big toe has been pushed out of alignment for years, the muscular arch under the inside of your foot flattens and weakens. Flat arches cause problems not only for your feet, but also for your ankles, knees, hips, and even back, since all parts are connected and depend on one another to work correctly and efficiently.

The soles of your shoes should be flexible, both lengthwise and from side to side. With each step, the human foot is supposed to roll from the heel to sole to toe. If shoes are inflexible, the natural roll is impossible, so the muscles, tendons, and joints of the feet can't work properly. This can lead to fallen arches and ankle problems.

Shoes with built-in arch supports work well if they actually fit your foot correctly. If not, they'll just rub against your foot and create friction. If you have high arches, flat feet, or painful feet, make an appointment with a podiatrist for a custom insole. The podiatrist will make a mold of the bottom of your foot and create an insole to fit your foot exactly.

The most important way to help your feet is to get rid of any shoes that are causing problems and buy yourself some slightly longer, broad-toed, flat, flexible shoes. Yes, they can still look good, and your feet will love them.

Tight nylons and socks can squash all of the toes together and bend them under, causing hammertoes. After you put on socks or stockings, stretch the toe area to the side and wiggle your toes inside. This will create room for the toes to be straight.

You can save your joints a lot of wear and tear by putting cushioned insoles into your shoes to absorb the impact of walking, particularly on asphalt and cement. A good choice is a sorbothane insole, a thin, flat, rubbery insole that can be trimmed with scissors to fit your shoes. Look for them in sporting goods stores.

If you have weak or fallen arches, the following exercises will really help. In addition, do the Buttock Clencher in chapter seven, often through the day. Clenching the butt muscles together not only decreases a swayback, but lifts the arches of the foot. The contracting butt muscles would slightly rotate the thighbone outward if friction between the soles of your feet and the floor weren't preventing your feet from rotating outward. The rotary force is transmitted to your feet and the arches lift. Give it a try. Stand tall with your feet hip-width apart and toes pointing straight ahead. Press your big toes into the floor. Clench your butt—think of pinching the muscles together. Feel your lower back stretch and your arches pull up.

Lining Up Your Big Toes
Realigns big toes that are pointing in; strengthens the arch of the foot.

1. To ease your big toes into the proper alignment with the rest of your foot, place a cotton ball between each big toe and the neighboring toe. (If you find the cotton balls fall out during this exercise, you can tape them in place.) The cotton ball should be thick enough to straighten the big toe. You could also buy rubber toe separators at any pharmacy.

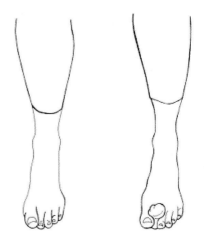

Big toe pulling in   Big tow aligned properly

2. Stand with your feet hip-width apart and your knees slightly bent. Press your big toes into the floor. At the same time, bend your knees and gently press them outward; when you look between your bent knees, you should be able to see your big toes. If you can't see your big toes, place your hands on the insides of your thighs and gently press your knees outward. Hold this position for a few seconds and then release. When you press the knees out, your big toes will want to come off the floor. Don't let them.

3. Repeat several times. You'll feel this in your arches.

Golden Arches

Strengthens the arches and ankles.

1. Place a cotton ball between your big toe and its neighboring toe. Holding on to the back of a chair for support, stand with your feet hip-width apart, head pulled back, rib cage lifted, abs tight.

2. Lift your heels off the floor, keeping your ankles straight. Don't let them bow out.

3. Lower your heels to the floor.

4. Breathe normally.

5. Repeat ten times. Gradually work your way up to fifty times.

High-Heel Blues

Stretches the Achilles tendons and calf muscles.

1. Stand with the balls of your feet on a book or the bottom stair of a staircase. Let your heels hang lower than the toes until you feel a good stretch in the back of your ankles.

2. Breath normally.

3. Hold for twenty seconds. Repeat several times throughout the day.

Helpful Hint

Consider seeing a podiatrist or sports medicine specialist to have your feet measured for orthotics. Orthotics are insoles made from a cast taken of the bottom of your feet. Your orthotics will address your specific foot and ankle issues. When placed in your shoes they will help keep your ankle joints properly aligned. Since your ankle bones are connected to your knees bones and your knee bones are connected to your hip bones, which are connected with your spinal bones, all of your joints can benefit from a well made, well fitting pair of orthotics.

Chapter 9

Total Posture Improvement Exercises

The following three strengthening exercises and two relaxation movements will make a big difference in your posture. Set aside a few minutes every day—like when watching the news—and do one or all. The reason they are so effective is that when lying down, gravity is off your spine and your head is lined up directly over your shoulders. In this position, you can strengthen all the muscles in your back, neck, and shoulders with your joints in good alignment, making these exercises extremely effective. Try them. You won't be disappointed.

Strengthening Exercises
Posture Press
Strengthens mid-back, back of shoulders, and abdominals. It reinforces good alignment.

1. Lie on your back, knees bent, feet flat on the floor.

2. Place arms at sides in a forty-five degree angle to torso.

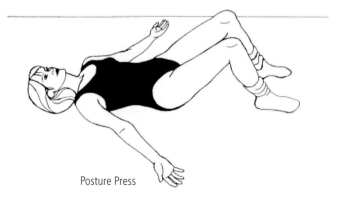

Posture Press

3. The palms of your hands need to face the ceiling.

4. Inhale. As you exhale, gently, press your lower back towards floor. Don't force anything. Then press your mid-back into floor, then your upper back. Think of pressing your whole spine, gently, into floor.

5. Next, press the back of your shoulders into the floor. As you do this, you should feel every muscle in your back contract.

6. Hold for a count of ten without holding your breath, then relax.

Triangle Press

Strengthens the muscles of the back, shoulders, and abdomen. It also stretches front of shoulders and chest.

1. Lie on the floor, knees bent, feet flat on floor.

2. Clasp your hands behind your head.

3. Press your shoulders away from your ears.

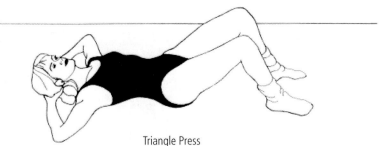

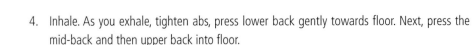

Triangle Press

4. Inhale. As you exhale, tighten abs, press lower back gently towards floor. Next, press the mid-back and then upper back into floor.

5. Next, press elbows into the floor. Feel your back muscles contract.

6. Hold this position for a slow count of ten without holding your breath. Then relax and repeat.

The Goal Post

Helps unround shoulders; strengthens mid/upper back and abdominals.

1. Lie on your back, knees bent, feet flat.

2. Place your arms in a goal post position.

3. Inhale. As you exhale, tighten abs and gently press your lower back towards the floor. Next, press your mid-back, then upper back into floor.

4. Slide your arms along the floor. First, slide your elbows towards your sides several inches. Then slide the arms back up. The whole time you are moving your arms, keep all of your back in contact with the floor.

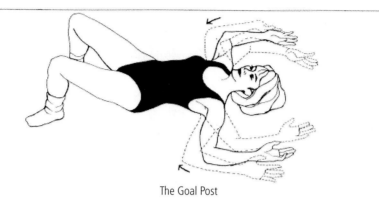

The Goal Post

Relaxation Movements

Do these stretches in between the Total Posture Improvement Exercises to help relax back muscles.

Mid-back Relaxer

1. Lie on the floor, knees bent, feet flat.
2. Clasp your hands and stretch your arms towards ceiling.
3. Draw big, easy circles—five times in one direction and then five times in the other.
4. Breathe normally.

Feel all the muscles in your back, especially between your shoulder blades, relax. This is like a gentle massage for the mid-back joints.

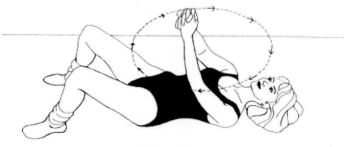

Mid-back Relaxer

Spine Stretch

Stretches the length of the spine.

1. Lie on your back, knees bent and feet flat on floor.

2. Stretch your arms behind your head and clasp them.

3. Swing your arms over your torso and clasp your right knee.

4. Pull your knee towards your chest. Hold this position for a few seconds without holding your breath. Uncurl and change sides. Alternate knees eight to ten times.

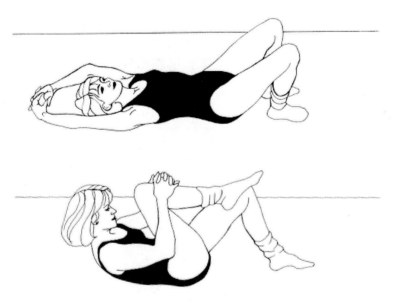

Spine Stretch

Helpful Hint

Make a point of doing these every day. If you regularly watch the news at night, get on the floor and do a few while watching the news or your favorite television show. If you've been working or doing any activity that had you in an awkward position, take a minute and do a few. They will feel really good because they will counteract and relieve any uneven tension in your muscles.

Chapter 10

Anywhere/Anytime Exercises

You probably are familiar with most of these Anywhere/Anytime Exercises because most are taken from previous problem-solving chapters. I've decided they need a chapter of their own because of the ease with which they can be performed throughout the day.

They are simple, mostly inconspicuous, tension-releasing exercises that require no change of clothes, no loss of time, and no perspiration. They can be done whenever you have a few moments: waiting at a red light or elevator, working at your desk or computer, talking on the phone, cooking, waiting in line, walking by a door frame, and so on. They will help you achieve the better and faster posture improvement results. These easy exercises will train your body to recognize proper alignment. They will strengthen weak muscles and stretch tight ones. They will help you look and feel better.

Try to sprinkle them often throughout your day, especially the ones that focus on your particular posture problems. It would be better to do a few posture improvement exercises every now and then throughout your day, and realign yourself every time you catch yourself slumping, than it would be to set aside thirty to sixty minutes, several times a week. If you exercised one hour each day, but spent the other twenty-three hours in poor alignment, you'll only get so far. Let these Anywhere/Anytime Exercises help you progress faster. You'll be amazed at how much exercise you can fit into your daily routine.

#1: Neck Glide (from chapter four)

Helps realign head over shoulders; helps relieve neck strain.

1. While standing or sitting, simply pull your head back over the middle of your shoulders. Think of trying to touch an imaginary wall with the back of your neck (not the back of your head or your neck will arch away from the wall).

2. Hold for ten seconds and relax. Do this whenever you realize your head has been hanging forward for a while, i.e., after reading or leaning over your desk, etc.

#2: Shoulder Blade Squeeze

Strengthens the muscles between the shoulder blades and mid-back.

1. Lift rib cage. Think of pulling up with your midsection.

2. Press your shoulder blades back towards your spine, and then press them down towards waistline.

3. Hold for a slow count of ten without holding your breath. Repeat often.

#3: The Hitchhiker (from chapter six)

Realigns shoulder joints; strengthens back of shoulder and stretches front of chest.

1. Whenever you realize your shoulders are rounding forward, lift your rib cage.

2. Externally rotate your arms until thumbs are pointing out, as if hitchhiking with both hands.

3. Press shoulder down, away from ears. Bend your elbows slightly.

4. Press arms back in little movements, from ten to twenty times. Concentrate on squeezing your shoulder blades together. Then relax.

#4: Elbow Press (from chapter four)

Strengthens back and chest muscles.

1. Lift your rib cage, relax your shoulders.

2. Place hands behind your head. Don't lace your fingers. Gently press the back of your head into your hands. Feel the muscles down the length of your spine tighten.

3. Hold for five to ten seconds and release.

4. Next, press your elbows back ten times. The elbows won't move very far. Concentrate on squeezing your shoulder blades towards each other.

5. Relax by clasping your hands in front of your chest. Stretch your arms forward and feel a stretch between the shoulder blades.

#5: Abdominal Tightener

Strengthens all four layers of abdominal muscles.

1. Inhale deeply. Feel your rib cage expand.

2. Exhale, through your mouth, as if blowing air through a straw.

3. As you exhale, pull your belly button towards your spine, as if you were trying to zip up a really tight pair of pants. Also, try to feel the bottom of your rib cage pull in.

4. Hold abs in, without holding your breath, for a slow count of ten. Slowly build up to thirty seconds.

5. To make this exercise even more powerful, at the end of your exhale, try to push a little more air out, and then a little more. You should feel all the muscles at the bottom of your rib cage and abdomen tighten even more. Relax and repeat.

#6: Buttock Clencher (from chapter seven)

Strengthens the abdominal muscles, stretches the lower back, and strengthens the buttock muscles.

1. Whenever you get a chance, clench your butt muscles and tighten your abs. Feel your pelvis go into a pelvic tilt. You should feel your lower back stretch.

2. Hold muscles clenched for ten to twenty seconds, without holding your breath. Relax.

#7: Spine Stretch (from chapter seven)

Elongates the spine. Can be done standing or sitting.

1. Lift up from your midsection. Think of separating your hipbones from your ribs.

2. Pull your abs in.

3. Breathe normally and practice walking with your midsection elongated.

#8: Deep Breathing Exercise (from chapter five)

Helps relax muscles whenever you feel tense.

1. Inhale through your nose. Think of inhaling into any area of muscle tightness, whether it is in your upper back or sides of neck or lower back.

2. When you exhale, consciously relax the tight muscle. Think of exhaling all the tension out with your breath.

#9: Door Frame Stretch (from chapter six)

Stretches the front of the shoulders and chest.

1. Whenever you get the opportunity, stand in a doorway.
2. Stretch your arms out at shoulder level. Bend your elbows at a ninety-degree angle. Fingers point toward ceiling, palms on door frame.
3. Tuck pelvis under by tightening abs.
4. Lean body forward until you feel a stretch in the front of your shoulders.
5. Hold for ten seconds without holding your breath.

#10: Wall Push-Up (from chapter four)

Helps align spine.

1. Stand with your back against a wall. Heel should be about six inches from the wall.
2. Let your arms hang by your sides with your palms facing forward.
3. Bend your knees slightly and gently, press the small of your back towards wall. Next, gently press mid-back, then upper back into wall.
4. Gently press the back of your neck towards wall. *Don't force anything*. Do this gently.
5. Last, press the back of your shoulders against the wall and feel the muscles in your back and shoulders contract and tighten.
6. Hold this position for ten seconds without holding your breath, then relax.

#11: Mid-back and Shoulder Strengthener (from chapter five)

Strengthens the muscles in mid-back and back of shoulders.

1. Make sure your bottom touches the back of the seat. Lift rib cage and relax shoulders. Have your back make full contact with the backrest.
2. Press the back of your shoulders into the backrest.
3. Hold for ten seconds without holding your breath. Feel all the muscles in your mid-back and back of shoulders contract.

#12: Chair Press Abdominal Strengthener

Here's another way to fit some abdominal strengthening into your day.

1. Make sure your bottom touches the back of the seat. Lift rib cage and relax shoulders. Have your back make full contact with the backrest.
2. Gently press your mid- and lower back into the backrest. You should feel your abs tighten. If this feels okay, press a little harder. (If you feel any pressure or discomfort in your lower back, stop.)
3. Hold for ten seconds or so without holding your breath then relax.

#13: Abdominal Stabilizer For Car Passengers

Strengthens all four layers of abdominal muscle.

1. Slide your bottom back until it touches the back of the car seat. Lift rib cage and relax shoulders.

2. There should be some space between your mid- and upper back and the car seat.

3. Secure your seat belt.

4. As the car moves, try to keep your torso perfectly still. You will feel your abs work hard to keep your torso from swaying as the car moves.

5. See if you can keep your torso from moving for thirty seconds. Build up to several minutes.

Helpful Hint

The more often you do these throughout the day, the quicker you will begin to reap the rewards of your new and improved posture. Not only will they help you look better, they can help rid you of annoying aches and pains.

Part III

Good Posture All Day Long

Chapter 11

The ABCs of Computer Comfort

We have become a nation of professional sitters. In offices all around America, people are sitting behind computers in really bad posture positions— necks craning forward, slumping upper backs, rounded shoulders.

Sitting for a long time is a major cause of back discomfort: it puts continuous pressure on the muscles and disks of the lower back. You may think your back muscles get a rest when you sit. Actually, they're working very hard to hold you upright. *Sitting puts 40 percent more pressure on the lower back disks than standing does.*

Sitting is particularly hard on the lower back if you sit with your lower back rounded out (called forward flexion). Make sure you sit with your pelvis in neutral: The top of the pelvic bones (iliac crests) should line up with the pubic bones. This is much less stressful for your lower back. Leaning over a desk and looking up and down from a keyboard to a computer screen puts pressure on the neck and upper back, too. By stopping the slouch, supporting your back properly, and avoiding the head-forward position, you will be able to work more comfortably and productively.

> **Teamwork**
> You can increase your awareness of your posture by enlisting the help of a friend at work. Ask him or her to let you know when your posture is bad. Do this for each other.

Replacing or modifying your office furniture is a good start. Fortunately, more manufacturers are producing furniture and accessories with good posture in mind. Ergonomically designed furniture can help reduce the user's fatigue and discomfort, and help increase productivity. Keep in mind that a piece of furniture is ergonomically correct for you only if it fits your particular body.

In any case, furniture alone can't help your posture. You also have to become more aware of how you sit, and you need to take little breaks during the day.

Setting Up a Desktop Computer Workstation

Try to make as many of the following adjustments to your desk and chair as possible. They will take away most of the causes of back and neck discomfort.

Monitors

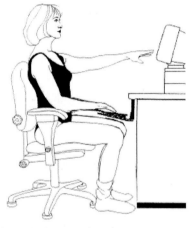

Sitting properly at the computer

- Your monitor should be about twelve to twenty-four inches away from your eyes.
- Your eyes should be level with the top of the monitor. This will let your eyes fall comfortably on the screen. Your head will be balanced over your spine, not tilted forward or backward. If your screen it too low, put it on a computer base or on books. If your screen is too high, lower it.
- The monitor should be placed directly in front of you–not to the left or right where you have to twist your spine or neck to see it.

Document Holder

- Using a document holder can eliminate uncomfortable neck twisting. Use the in-line document holder that sits between the keyboard and tray. Put your work at eye level without having to twist your neck or spine. You want to tilt the angle of your work—not the angle of your head on your neck.

Bifocals/Progressive Lens Wearers

- Your chair should recline to 110 degrees instead of 90 degrees.
- Slightly tilt your monitor back by placing something under the front edge of the monitor. This should allow you to view the screen comfortably without craning your neck forward or tilting your head back too far.

Keyboard Surface

- The perfect keyboard level for you is at elbow level, with your forearms in a ninety-degree angle with your upper arm or slightly lower with the keyboard base gently sloped away from the user. This position allows the back, neck, shoulders, and arms to relax more. If your keyboard level is too low, place blocks under the legs of the desk. If it's too high, raise your chair seat and use a footrest.

Using a Mouse

- Your mouse needs to be as close to you as possible.

- When using it, your elbow should be at a ninety-degree angle to your forearm.

- Keep upper arm relaxed and close to your body.

- Check office supply stores for mouse pads that attach to the arm of your chair. Over-reaching for a mouse causes the spine to twist slightly. This means that within seconds, there'll be more tension on one side of your spine than the other.

Computer Chair

- The ideal computer chair has adjustable armrests that support your arms at elbow level. Both the width and height of the rests should be adjustable. By supporting your elbows on an armrest, 25 percent of the pressure load is taken off the lower back disks. Armrests also take the burden of holding up the arms from the mid- and upper back muscles.

- The ideal chair will support the width and length of your back. At the very least, the chair back should reach to your shoulder blades.

Retrofitting a Chair

If you can't buy a new chair, try these inexpensive ways to adjust the seat height, back support, and armrests.

- If the seat is too low and the armrests are too high, place a cushion on the seat to raise your body. Use a telephone book or box as a stool for your feet.

- If the chair depth was made for a person with longer legs, place a cushion between the chair back and your body.

- If you don't have armrests, try placing a box on your lap and resting your elbows on it.

- To prevent your lower back from slouching backward, place a small lumbar pillow behind you to remind you to sit with your pelvis in neutral.

- The back of the chair, the chair rest, should be fairly straight; at a 90- to 110-degree angle to the seat.

- When you sit, make sure you slide your bottom all the way to the back of the chair seat. Your buttocks and the middle of your back should make contact with the backrest.

- The chair seat should be padded with rounded edges and slightly tilted. The back of the seat should be slightly lower than the front, so the buttocks can be placed against the back of the chair and the knees can be slightly higher than the hips.

- Your knees should extend no more than a few inches from the edge of the seat.

- The chair seat should be long enough to support the whole length of your thighs. That way, the weight of your body is evenly distributed over your buttocks and the full length of your thighs. If the seat is not long enough to support the length of your thighs, you'll end up crossing your legs, which causes imbalances in the hips and lower back. Sitting with your legs crossed also can contribute to varicose veins and poor circulation.

- Your feet should rest flat on the floor. Adjust the height of the seat or get a footrest. A telephone book works in a pinch.

- Your chair should swivel and be on casters so you can adjust your reach and line of vision without twisting, bending, or leaning forward.

> **Sitting Too Much?**
> Sitting too long without moving around is a major contributor to back pain in office workers. Here are some ways you can sit less and stand more.
> - Stand when you're talking on the phone.
> - Walk over to a colleague's desk instead of phoning or E-mailing.
> - Position equipment so you'll have to stand and walk; for example, put the printer or fax across the room.
> - To increase circulation, clench and release your buttock muscles.
> - Shift positions often to change the load on your spine.

Avoiding Carpal Tunnel Syndrome

Flexing your wrists while doing repetitive hand and finger movements, such as typing or working a cash register, places you at higher risk for developing carpal tunnel syndrome: numbness, tingling, burning, or pain in the middle and index fingers and thumb (and sometimes all the fingers). Eventually, your hand grip may weaken. Carpal tunnel syndrome is increasingly common among office workers. You can reduce your risk by modifying your workstation and changing the way you use your hands.

Hand and finger movements repeated over and over for a long time, especially when the wrists are lower than the fingers, cause inflammation around the median nerve, which runs through a narrow tunnel of bone and ligament in the middle of the wrist. Since bones and ligaments have no give, this puts pressure on the nerve and causes the symptoms.

If you have any of the above-mentioned symptoms, see your doctor for diagnosis and treatment. Early intervention can help prevent and minimize symptoms. Stop the problem before it becomes severe.

If you work at a keyboard, and especially if it causes you discomfort, also try to make the following changes at work:

- Your keyboard should be at elbow level or a little lower. If the keyboard base slopes gently away from you, your hands will be a little lower than your wrists. Research from Cornell University shows this position puts less stress on nerves and soft tissue. Make sure your wrists are not flexed with the fingers higher than the wrists. Bending the wrist this way narrows the tunnel through which the median nerve passes, so it can actually contribute to carpel tunnel syndrome or even worsen the problem.

- Rest your hands periodically throughout the day.

- If you can, rotate work activities so you don't spend hours at a time at the keyboard.

- Exercises that strengthen the hand and arm muscles may help. When these muscles are weak, there's a tendency to compensate with poor wrist position.

- If you are experiencing the symptoms of carpal tunnel syndrome, a physical therapist can design splints for you to wear while you work, which protect your wrists and keeps them in a neutral position. The splints will be specific to the kind of work you do. You may want to wear a wrist splint at night. It will keep your wrist in a neutral position so symptoms don't wake you. It may also reduce your symptoms during the daytime.

Laptop Tips

Laptops are fast becoming the most popular way to do computer work. They can be great for short periods of work. Laptops are convenient, but can be extremely hard on your back and neck. Using a laptop is always a trade-off between poor head and neck posture and poor hand and wrist posture. Because of their design, you will either get the screen level correct for your body or the keyboard level correct—never both.

If you spend hours on your laptop, you may consider purchasing the following:

- an external monitor,
- an external keyboard, preferably with a negative tilt,
- a docking station.

Occasional users should:

- Find a chair that is comfortable and that reclines back 110 degrees.
- Position laptop in your lap for the most neutral wrist posture.
- Angle the screen to be seen with the least amount of neck deviation.

Full-time users should:

- Position laptop on desk in front of you so you can see the screen without bending your neck. You may need to elevate the laptop off the desk using a monitor pedestal.
- Separate the keyboard and mouse.
- Connect a separate keyboard and mouse to back of laptop. A negative tilt keyboard is preferable to ensure a neutral wrist posture. Use a mouse platform to raise the mouse off the desk.

For a Desk Without a Computer

The same features of a good chair apply if you work at a desk without a computer. The top of the desk should be at elbow level.

Angling the surface of your workstation prevents you from having to lean over your work. Constantly leaning the head forward over a desk causes much back and neck misery. Office supply stores sell inexpensive drafting boards that can be placed on top of a desk. You can also prop up a clipboard. Adjust the surface so you are looking straight ahead rather than down. A raised work surface will enable you to sit and work with your back and head straight and balanced. You could also tilt the desk surface toward you by putting books or boards under the back legs of the desk. Propping up your work surface, however you can, will allow you to work with your head directly over your spine.

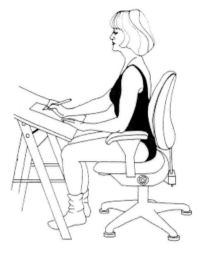

Tilting a desk surface

The way you talk on the phone can cause posture problems, too. Don't clench your phone receiver between your ear and shoulder. If you need to keep your hands free, get a wireless headset.

Desk Exercises and Stretches

You can do these exercises right at your desk. They'll relieve stress in both your body and mind. Work them in throughout the day. Also, take a one-minute break to stand up and stretch once an hour.

Exhale and Relax

Relaxes muscles whenever you feel tense.

1. Inhale through your nose. Think of inhaling into the tight muscle, whether it is your upper back or sides of neck or lower back.

2. When you exhale, consciously relax the tight muscle. Exhale all of the tension.

3. Repeat several times.

Back Lift

Strengthens the muscles of the lower back.

1. Sit on the edge of a chair. Clasp your hands behind your head.

2. Bend forward as far as you comfortably can. Then slowly lift your head and torso until your back and neck are at a forty-five-degree angle to the floor. As you lift, squeeze your shoulder blades together.

3. Repeat eight times.

Back Lift

Total Body Stretches

1. Raise your shoulders toward your ears, and then press them down as far as possible. Hold for five to ten seconds. Repeat twice.

2. Circle your shoulders, five times in one direction, five times in the other.

3. Squeeze your shoulder blades together, then press them down. Hold for a count of five without holding your breath then relax. Repeat three times.

4. Clasp your hands behind your head. Relax and drop your shoulders. Press your elbows back, squeezing your shoulder blades together. Hold for five seconds, then relax. Repeat three times.

5. Clasp your hands behind your waist. Slowly lift your clasped hands away from your body. Feel your chest muscles stretch and your shoulder blades pull toward one another. Hold for five seconds and relax. Repeat three times.

6. Take a deep breath and feel your rib cage expand. As you exhale, tighten your abdominals as much as possible. Pull them in as if you were trying to zip up a really tight pair of pants. Hold the muscles tight for a slow count of five, then relax. Repeat several times.

7. Spend a few seconds doing the Shoulder Straightener in chapter six.

Helpful Hints

- Always set up your computer workstation for back and neck comfort.
- Take breaks often.
- Get up and walk around every hour or so.
- Take the stairs instead of the elevator.
- Stand when on the phone.
- Take one-minute exercise breaks several times each day.

Chapter 12

Planes, Trains, and Automobiles

Whether you travel by plane, train, or automobile, sitting in confined spaces for long periods can cause a number of problems–considerable pressure on joints, crimped circulation, increased risk of blood clots, stiff, cramped muscles, increased fatigue, back and neck pain, and knee discomfort.

Travel Tips for Planes and Trains

Good posture/body mechanics is the key to prevention of back, neck, and joint discomfort when traveling.

- Make frequent posture changes: get up every forty-five minutes or so to walk or stand.
- Adjust the seat as best you can to an upright position.
- Slide your butt back until it touches the back of the seat.
- If there's a big space between your lower back and chair seat, use a lumbar pillow or rolled up sweater and place it behind your back.
- Use a traveler's pillow to decrease neck strain when snoozing.
- If your feet don't touch the floor, place a backpack or carry-on on the floor.
- Shift weight frequently to reduce prolonged pressure on any given point.
- Hips and knees should be at ninety-degree angles.
- Keep shoulders relaxed in line with trunk and upper back to allow even loading through spine.
- Let forearms and elbows rest on armrests.
- If armrests are too low or hard, use a small pillow under each forearm.

Travel Exercises
Feet and Ankles
- Circle feet in one direction then the other.
- Pump feet by lifting heels, keeping toes on floor.
- Pump feet like pushing on a car accelerator.
- Tap toes like windshield wiper blades on a car. Keep your heels on the floor and tap toes from left to right.

Torso
- Inhale, pull oxygen down to bottom of rib cage. Feel chest expand. Exhale and pull abdominals in.
- Reach arms towards ceiling and stretch upwards.
- Turn body and head to look over right shoulder and then left.

Shoulders/Upper Back
- Press shoulder blades back towards spine and then down towards waist.
- Shrug and circle shoulders.
- Lift shoulders towards back of head, then press them down.

Head/Neck
- Press neck to back of chair rest.
- Stick chin forward, then pull it back (think of a turtle pulling its head back into its shell).
- Turn head towards right shoulder then left.

Luggage Lifting Tips
- Bend knees and use thigh muscles–don't lean over from waist.
- Before lifting, pull abdominals in as tightly as possible.
- Pivot with feet, don't twist spine.
- Carry heavy items close to body.
- Switch shoulders often, if carrying a shoulder bag.
- Place luggage or briefcase in back seat of car from back door. Don't get in front seat and then twist to retrieve or place things in the back seat. If you have a two-door car, place luggage in the trunk, not the back seat.

Travel Tips for Automobiles

We all spend a lot of time coming and going in our cars. Most of the time, we're slumped over the wheel. The next time you're waiting for a red light, look into the nearby cars. The drivers' heads will probably be hanging forward, their upper backs rounded over. This position not only contributes to poor posture in general, but is also tiring during a long drive. Good posture can help a driver stay comfortable and alert.

Adjusting Your Car Seat

You can adjust your seat so it will help keep your body properly aligned while you drive. All these little adjustments will make a big difference in your posture and comfort.

- Move the seat close enough to the pedals and steering wheel that your knees are bent and your bottom rests against the back of seat. If the seat is too far away from the pedals, you will not be able to sit with your pelvis in neutral or with your bottom against the seat back. However, for air bag safety, you should be at least thirteen inches away from steering wheel.

- You want to be able to rest against the back of the seat and still sit up straight. Bring your seat to its straightest position. Ideally, it should incline no more than 110 degrees.

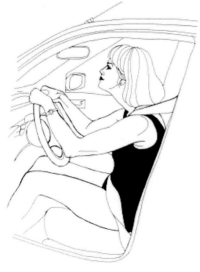

Look familiar?

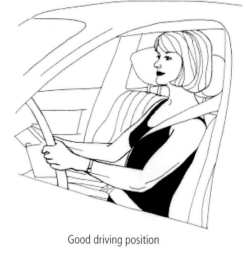

Good driving position

- Adjust the headrest so you can sit with the back of your head resting against it. This position puts your head directly over your spine and allows your neck muscles to relax while you drive. It is also safer in case you are rear-ended. When the headrest sits at neck level, your head can snap back over it in a collision. If your car's headrest tilts too far back, make it thicker by attaching a rolled-up towel with rubber bands.

- In driver education classes we all learned to hold the steering wheel in the ten o'clock and two o'clock positions. This encourages the driver to round the shoulders and raise the shoulders and arms, causing unnecessary tension in the shoulder and neck muscles. Instead, get a lower grip on the steering wheel, at nine o'clock and three o'clock. In this position, the upper arms hang more vertically and the shoulders are less hunched, which allows the neck muscles to relax, greatly reducing discomfort and fatigue.

> **Car Shopping**
>
> Many cars have seats that are too low, too soft, and too slanted. After several minutes of driving, the back and legs become very uncomfortable. Next time you're shopping for a car, investigate the following:
>
> - How straight can you get the backrest?
> - Is the headrest adjustable? Can it reach your head or only the back of your neck?
> - Does the headrest push your head forward too much?
> - Is the seat long enough to support fully the weight of both your thighs, especially the accelerator leg? (This distributes the body's weight over a wider area and prevents fatigue.)
> - Is the seat at the right height (or is it adjustable)?
> - Is the seat back too slanted? Does it cause you to lean too far back when leaning against it? Seats that aren't straight enough do not allow you to sit correctly.
> - Is the seat too soft? Does it sag in the center, causing your hips to roll to one side? A seat that is too soft allows you to slump and slouch.

Car Exercises

All those trips in your car are opportunities to build some posture work into your daily routine. Talk about turning things around–your car can help your posture instead of harming it.

The following exercises can be done while you're stopped at red lights. Don't try to do them while you're driving. They will help strengthen the mid- and upper back and abdominals. If you're on a long trip, they'll refresh you, too–do them at the rest area or when you stop for lunch. If you're a passenger, you can exercise while you're rolling along.

- Lift up your rib cage and press the back of your head against the headrest. Stay lifted that way while you drive.

- Press the back of your shoulders into the seat as if you were trying to bring your shoulder blades closer together. Hold for ten seconds without holding your breath then relax. Repeat several times.

- Tighten your abdominals. Take a deep breath. As you exhale, pull your belly button toward your spine and hold for ten seconds. See if you can feel the bottom of your rib cage pull in. Don't hold your breath. Gradually build up to holding the abdominals for thirty seconds.

- Lengthen your midsection. Pretend your spine is growing longer. Think of pulling your rib cage away from your hipbones. Pull your abdominals in snugly. See how long you can maintain this elongation at red lights.

- Hug yourself by placing your hands on the opposite shoulders. While you keep your hands on your shoulders, press your elbows forward and round your upper back to stretch the muscles between your shoulder blades.

Helpful Hint

Sit in your car with proper alignment as described above. Adjust your rear view mirror so you can see perfectly through it. You'll know you are slumping while driving if, when you look in your rear view mirror, you have to adjust it to see behind you properly.

Chapter 13

Sleeping

I f you've ever woken up feeling like you were run over by a truck, you know
that posture matters when you're sleeping, too. Certain sleeping positions
can intensify a swayback or give you a pain in the neck. Considering that you
spend about a third of your life sleeping, your position can make a big difference in your overall posture as well as the comfort of your nights and morn-
ings.

Most people who get an aching back while sleeping assume the problem
is their mattress. Unless the mattress is lumpy or sags one way or the other, it
doesn't matter as much as the position in which you sleep. The most important
thing is to keep your head level with your spine. Often the solution is a few
well-placed pillows. Proper support of the body can take a lot of stress off the
joints of the spine.

Sleeping on Your Side

The side is a good sleeping position, but it creates the widest gap between your
neck and the mattress. Side sleepers need a firm pillow that provides lots of
support for the neck. Foam pillows give more support than cushy down ones.
The pillow or pillows should be as wide as the distance from your ear to the

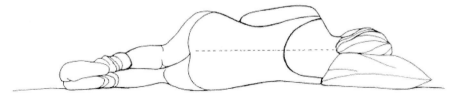

Spine straight

Sleeping 93

end of your shoulder. If the pillows aren't high enough, your head will tilt down toward the mattress and your shoulder will really roll under—not good if you already tend to have rounded shoulders. Your pillow has to be wide enough to support your head and keep it in neutral (that is, level with your spine), but not so wide that it tilts your head toward the ceiling. Ask your significant other or a friend to check your sleeping position.

When you lie on your side with your knees stacked on top of one another, the weight of the top thigh pulls on the joints in the lower spine and the hip socket. You can take the pressure off by placing a regular-size bed pillow between your knees and lower legs. You'll find this extremely comfortable, especially if you have lower back or hip discomfort. If you roll to your other side during the night, your body will soon learn to take the pillow along.

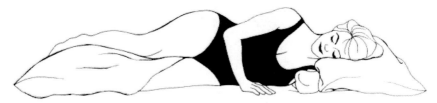

Place a pillow between your legs.

Sleeping on Your Back

Back sleepers should put a pillow or rolled-up beach towel under their lower legs. When the lower legs are elevated, the lower back is in a more stretched position, which takes pressure off the spinal joints. Because of the way the leg bone fits into the hip socket, when you lie down with your legs straight out, the curve in the lower back is accentuated. This puts pressure on spinal nerves, soft tissue, and joints. You could wake up with a very sore, stiff back.

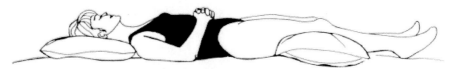

Pillow placement for sleeping on your back

If your head tends to hang forward, the last thing you want to do is sleep with two or three pillows lifting your head beyond your shoulders all night.

Your neck should stay in a neutral position, level with your spine. When you're lying on your back, your face should be parallel to the ceiling. Your head should not be pushed forward or allowed to roll back, making the neck too arched and the chin jut forward.

The goal is to sleep with one thin, flat pillow that allows correct alignment. If you are used to sleeping on your back with several pillows, take one pillow away at a time so you can gradually get used to the new height.

Sleeping on Your Stomach

Sleeping on your stomach can be extremely hard on your neck and lower back. You have to turn your head to one side or the other, which puts a lot of pressure on the neck. Stomach sleeping allows the lower back to sag into the mattress.

A small pillow or rolled-up towel can prevent your lower back from sagging.

If you are one of those people who can only sleep on their stomach, place a small pillow or rolled-up towel under your abdomen to prevent the lower back from sagging down. For even greater back relief, sleep with one knee bent toward your chest. Make sure the pillow under your head is as flat as possible so your neck doesn't have to arch as well as twist to one side.

Buying a Mattress

You need a new mattress if one or more of the following is true.

- Your current mattress is more than ten years old and hasn't been flipped or turned every couple of months.
- Your mattress has lumps or it sags into the middle.
- You can feel the springs or coils.
- You continually wake up with a sore, stiff back or neck.
- You roll into your partner during the night.

When you're buying a mattress, don't be shy—lie down on the models you're considering and stay in your most common sleep position for at least fifteen minutes. Select a mattress that is comfortable for you. Firm mattresses usually support the spine better, but whether the mattress is extra firm, firm, or medium soft is a matter of personal preference. A mattress that is too soft will let your body sag, causing you to wake up with aches and pains. Going from a soft mattress to a firm one will take some getting used to, and your back may be sore for the first week. Soon your body will get used to it, however, and in the long run your spine will be better supported while you sleep. If your current mattress is too soft, but otherwise still good, you can add support by placing a three-quarters-of-an-inch-thick piece of plywood between the mattress and the box spring.

Pillow Talk

There are many kinds of pillows on the market today—rolls in all different shapes and sizes, contoured pillows, pillows stuffed with down and synthetics. Your pillow's job is to keep your neck in neutral and your head level with your spine. It should not push your head forward, allow your neck to arch, or tilt your head to the left or right.

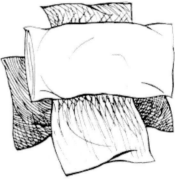

- Side sleepers need firm pillows to fill the wide gap between the neck and mattress.

- Back sleepers need soft pillows that allow the head to sink in, so it's not pushed too far forward.

- Stomach sleepers need a thin, flat pillow or no pillow at all.

- Contoured pillows are especially designed to support the neck whether you sleep on your back or your side. They have an indentation in the middle so the head is not pushed forward. They are raised on the ends, to support the neck if the person rolls onto either side. If you tend to change position during the night, a contoured pillow is a good choice.

- If you rest, read, or watch TV in bed, you don't want to thrust your head forward. Instead, stack up the pillows to raise your torso from the waist.

Helpful Hint

Statistics say we move every eleven minutes during sleep. My hunch is if we are moving that much, it is because our joints are uncomfortable.

Mattress toppers help with sleeping comfort by making your joints more comfortable. They help distribute your pressure points—points of contact with the mattress—more evenly and can take a considerable amount of pressure off your joints. A few strategically placed pillows and a good mattress topper can make a world of difference in joint comfort.

The least expensive type of mattress topper is the one that resembles the inside of an egg crate. It has a series of raised, foam ridges that distribute the pressure on body parts more evenly, allow for better circulation, and keep you cooler by allowing air to pass below you. There are many high tech mattress toppers available now for considerably more money. Some are made of feathers, some of lambskin, and some of memory foam.

Chapter 14

Lifting Safely

Think about all the things you lift in a day: groceries, children, suitcases, vacuum cleaner, laundry basket, garbage, tools, furniture... Perhaps your job involves lifting: roof shingles, furniture, mail, groceries, hospital patients... Do you just reach out and hoist the load? In a quick second, you can hurt your back and cause yourself much misery. You need to stop and think about how you are lifting.

Lifting puts tremendous pressure on your vertebrae, and the way that you lift an object makes a huge difference. According to Dr. I. A. Kapandji, in his book *The Physiology of the Joints*, lifting a twenty-pound object with your knees flexed and trunk vertical exerts about 300 pounds of force on the vertebrae. Lifting the same weight while keeping the knees straight and bending over from the waist exerts about *560 pounds* on the spine (almost twice as much).

To protect your back, learn and practice good lifting techniques. If you do a lot of lifting in your work or daily life, you should also do exercises to strengthen your abdominal muscles. Strong abs can reduce compression of the disks in your spine by as much as 50 percent.

Lifting Techniques

To keep your back working smoothly, you need to lift objects correctly. Safe lifting techniques can save your back from accidental strain and overload.

- Before you lift something, always judge its weight by pushing it with your foot. If it seems too heavy, divide the load or get someone to help you. Never carry anything you can't manage with ease.

- *Never try to pick something up when your torso is twisted.* Lifting while the spine is twisted causes the majority of lifting injuries. Instead, turn to face the object. Be sure your knees and torso are facing in the same direction.

- If you need to turn while holding the object, for example to place it onto a table, turn your feet instead of your back. Keeping your torso straight, pivot on the balls of your feet. This way your whole body turns without your spine twisting.

- Get as close to the object as possible. The closer you are, the less strain there will be on the spine.

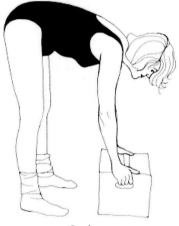

- Never bend from your waist. Bend your knees and hips instead. This lets the large muscles in your legs do most of the work. Bending from your waist to lift an object requires your back muscles to exert nearly twice the force.

Don't

- Tighten your abdominals as hard as you can to support your lower back before lifting or reaching for an object. When you pull your abdominals in, you increase intra-abdominal pressure, which decreases stress on your disks and joints by 50 percent. To tighten the abdominals, take a deep breath. When you exhale, pull your belly button toward your spine. Suck in as if you were trying to zip up a really tight pair of pants. Hold the abdominals in as you lift the object.

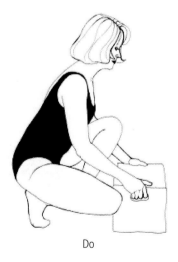

Do

Hold them in when putting the object down, too. Try not to hold your breath.

- Hold the object you've lifted close to your body as you gradually straighten your legs to a standing position. When carrying an object, keep your arms close to your rib cage. The further away from your body you hold a weight, the more the disks of the spine are compressed and the more the muscles have to work.

- When reaching for objects overhead, the same rules apply. Get as close to the object as possible. Face the object so your torso can be straight and not twisted and pull your abdominal muscles tight before you reach. Never lift a heavy object higher than your waist.

Lifting Tips

Many a person has toppled over with back pain after shoveling snow, raking the leaves, moving into a new house, even hoisting a heavy suitcase. These tips will help you lift things safely.

- Buy luggage with wheels. Don't try to carry heavy suitcases through the airport. It is almost impossible to balance the weight of a heavy suitcase evenly, and one side of your body ends up carrying the entire load.

- Try not to carry overloaded shopping bags. They place too much stress on your back, elbows, knees, and feet. Instead of carrying one very heavy shopping bag, distribute the groceries between two shopping bags, preferably with handles. Carry one in each hand.

- Moving heavy furniture can ruin your back. If possible, hire a professional mover.

- When vacuuming, never bend or twist your spine. When moving the wand forward or from side to side, use your leg muscles instead of your back— bend your knees slightly and shift your weight from one foot to another. Keep your arm close to your body rather than reaching to cover as much ground as possible.

- When raking leaves, bend your knees and place one foot forward; change the front foot often. Move forward or backward, shifting your weight from foot to foot, and dragging the leaves with the rake as you move. Don't reach too far in front of you with the rake.

- Shoveling snow can be extremely tough on the back. Take small steps; the job will take longer, but your back will be safer. Bend your knees when scooping. Before lifting the shovel filled with snow, tighten your abs to support your back. The further you try to throw the snow, the more you'll strain your back. Trade sides every few minutes. If you can afford it, a small snow thrower will make the job easier and save lots of wear and tear on your muscles and joints. Or hire a plow to take care of the driveway.

Helpful Hint

There will be times it's just not worth the risk of hurting your back. You have choices to enlist help—volunteer or paid—and making the correct choice for you pays off in the long run.

Chapter 15

Good Posture for Sports and Workouts

Working out or playing a sport can improve your posture by strengthening and stretching the muscles in your back, chest, abdomen, and legs. Regular aerobic and strengthening exercises can help your posture while they're making your heart and bones strong, increasing your oxygen flow, keeping your weight healthy, and reducing stress.

However, sports and workouts can strain, and even injure, your spine, joints, and muscles if you are not correctly aligned while you're doing them. If your upper back is curved too far forward, you can hurt your neck upper back or shoulders. If your lower back is swayed, you can have knee, hip, or lower-back injuries. Poor body alignment leads to joint instability, movement restriction, overuse injury, unnecessary wear and tear on joint tissue.

Good alignment is key. If you practice good posture, you'll not only reduce your chances of injury, but will enhance your athletic performance. You will have more grace, power, and breathing capacity. You'll reduce the risk of muscle pulls, tendon tears, joint injury, back pain, torn rotator cuff, bursitis, and osteoarthritis. Whatever sport you participate in, you need balanced joints and balanced strength on each side of your joint.

If you have already sustained an injury, wonderful resources that should be utilized are physical therapists, chiropractors, and personal trainers. Improving your posture will enhance the results, bring about quicker recovery with longer lasting results, and will decrease the chance of recurrence.

Posture and Biking

Biking is great aerobic exercise, but it's crucial that you choose the right bike and adjust it correctly.

- Select a bike frame that is the right size for your height and weight.

- Adjust the seat so when the pedal is farthest away from you, your leg is fully extended but your knee isn't locked back.

- Most important for good posture, adjust the handlebars so you don't have to lean far forward. It is better for your back to be sitting upright. Racing bikes with handlebars that curl downwards encourage a head-forward position, hunched upper back, and rounded shoulders. Plus, to see in front, you have to arch your neck. Mountain bikes and hybrids with straighter handlebars are better designed for the back. Many bike stores sell attachments to raise the grips of the handlebars.

Posture and Golf

Many people desperately want to improve their game. They spend lots of money on state-of-the art clubs to increase power behind their swing. What some fail to realize is that improving your posture/alignment can have the most impact on not only your swing but the power behind the swing.

Good Golfing Posture Tips

- Knees should be slightly flexed and directly over the balls of your feet for balance.

- The center of the upper spine, knees, and balls of feet should be stacked when viewed from behind the ball on the target line.

- Body should bend at the hips, not the waist.

- Your buttocks should protrude slightly.

- The spine is the axis of rotation for the swing, so it should be bent towards the ball from the hips at approximately a forty-five-degree angle to the shaft of the club.

- Your vertebrae should be in a straight line with no bending in the mid-back.

- If you slouch, every one degree of bend decreases shoulder turn by 1.5 degrees.

- Keep spine in line for longer drives and more consistent ball striking.

- Keep your chin up and your chest out to encourage a better shoulder turn.

If you are a golfer, your game will improve if you work on:

1. Strengthening the abdominals.

2. Paying extra attention stretching the tighter side and strengthening the weaker side. Do the Well-Balanced Golfer exercise (below).

3. Shoulder joint alignment.

4. Mid- and upper back alignment.

When carrying your golf bag, make sure the weight is evenly distributed across your back. Occasionally switch shoulders. Before lifting the bag, pull your abdominals in tightly to support the lower back. You might want to invest in a golf bag with wheels on the bottom, which can save your back a lot of stress and strain.

Well-Balanced Golfer
Prevents muscular imbalances caused by a golf swing.

1. Lie on the floor on your back, bend your knees, and place your feet on the floor about eighteen inches from your bottom. Place both hands behind your head. Tighten your abdominals.

2. If you always swing to the left, slowly lift your left shoulder and your right knee toward each other. Hold for a slow count of five as you pull your belly button into your spine. Release. Do the opposite if you swing to the right.

3. Repeat ten to twenty times.

Posture and Tennis

When playing tennis, squash, or handball, you have to be ready to move quickly in any direction at any moment. This requires very flexible hips. You can increase the range of motion of the hips by stretching your hips, quads, and hamstrings. Keeping these muscles stretched and flexible will reduce the chance of injury and increase your power and agility. See the exercises in chapter seven.

If you always swing your racquet to the same side, one side of your torso will become tight and contracted, the other weak and stretched. Practice the Sink Stretch in chapter seven and the Well-Balanced Golfer in this chapter.

Though you will have to twist and turn in these sports, try to avoid sudden or jerky motions.

Posture and Running

Running and jogging pound the body against hard road surfaces over and over again. This can injure the knees, ankles, hips, back, shins, Achilles tendons, and/or calf muscles. When running or jogging, you can reduce the shock to the body by striking the ground heel first. Roll from the heel to the little toe. Then roll from the outside to the inside of the foot and push off with the big toe. Keep your abdominal muscles pulled in to support your lower back.

Make sure your rib cage is lifted and your head is pulled back over your shoulders. Don't lead with your head or chest. Holding a balanced posture while running will work more muscles in your abdomen and upper body.

Runners need to stretch their hamstrings, quads, and Achilles tendons. See the stretches in chapter seven. To stretch the Achilles tendon, do the High Heel Blues exercise in chapter eight.

Posture and Weight Lifting

Most gyms and health clubs have a variety of state-of-the-art weight machines designed to keep your body in the correct position while you strengthen particular muscle groups. Gyms usually have fitness trainers who can help you begin a safe and effective program.

Proper alignment is essential when using strength training machines because poor form can set you up for joint and muscle injury. Here are some ways you can make your workouts at the gym safe and effective:

- Most weight machines are constructed to hold your body in the correct position while lifting. The joint you will be moving should be lined up with a hinge on the machine. Each time you use the machine, adjust the seat pads and other components to fit the size of your body.

- Have a personal trainer go through each machine with you to help you determine the correct machine settings for your body.

- The trainer can also help you determine the amount of weight you should be lifting. Your maximum is the amount of weight you can lift just once. Most people build up to working at 70 to 80 percent of their maximum strength. Start with low weights (50 to 60 percent of your maximum) until you get the hang of each machine.

- Warm up for five to ten minutes with light aerobic activity like cycling or walking on the treadmill.

- Whatever machine you use, always keep your head directly over your shoulders. Keep your rib cage lifted, your shoulder blades pulled back.

- Always tighten your abdominals before pushing or pulling the weight.

- If a padded backrest is provided for your back and head, use it. Sit tall with your back and head resting against the pad. This will keep your torso and head aligned.

- Always keep your shoulders squared and pressed away from your ears. If you find that your shoulders hunch toward your ears while using a machine, raise the seat slightly.

- Do the exercises slowly. There should be a three-second rest between each repetition.

- Always exhale when you pull the weights toward you or push them away from you.

- Don't hold your breath, as this increases the pressure in your chest, abdomen, and head.

- Don't lock your knees or elbows. This puts too much pressure on the joints, and can lead to injury.

- Drink water before, during, and after using machines. Even slight dehydration can affect the quality of your workout.

- Cool down afterward. Ask the trainer for appropriate stretches.

Good posture is also important if you use aerobic machines like StairMasters and treadmills. Many times I've seen people working really hard, but leaning forward to hold onto the handrails for dear life. They're reinforcing bad posture: forward head, slumped upper back. Instead, align yourself first by doing the One Minute To Better Posture technique. You'll not only be helping your posture, but you'll burn more calories, since you'll be using more muscles.

Posture and Walking

Walking is an excellent low-impact exercise. To make it a total body workout, always lift your rib cage up, pull your shoulder blades back, and press your shoulders away from your ears. If you tighten your abdominals while walking, the opposing movements of your arms and legs will help strengthen them.

Helpful Hint

Good athletic shoes that fit properly will help prevent injuries.

- Choose a shoe with cushioned insoles that will absorb shock and prevent the jarring of your joints. Replace the shoes (or insoles) when the insoles no longer spring back into shape after each step, even if the other parts of the shoes are still in good shape.

- Match your shoe to your activity. There are shoes designed to stabilize the foot and reduce the risk of injury during particular sports, including walking, running, aerobic dancing, and racquet sports.

- The upper part of the shoe should be flexible, but should also support the foot during movement.

- When selecting a size, stand on one foot at a time, wiggle your toes, and walk or run around the store a bit.

- The shoe has to be wide enough that the widest part of your foot fits comfortably. Shop late in the day, because feet swell during the day.

- When trying on shoes, wear the same kind of socks you will when exercising.

- If you get a pain across the top of your foot, your laces may be too tight. Loosen them to restore circulation.

Chapter 16

Hobbies and Crafting

If you enjoy any of the following activities—crafting, jewelry making, scrapbooking, sewing, needlepoint, crocheting, knitting, or decorative painting— you face some extra posture challenges.

The typical mechanical problems that crafters face include:

- long hours of sitting
- awkward positions involving arms, shoulders, wrists, neck, and lower back
- twisting, turning, reaching for tools
- hand tool use, especially plier use and filing, forces wrist out of its neutral position
- bad seating design
- slouching sitting posture
- crafting at incorrect working heights.

Therefore, crafters often exhibit these the following alignment problems:

- forward-head position
- stooping upper backs
- rounded shoulders
- tight, tense neck muscles
- carpel tunnel syndrome
- tight chest muscles

- aching lower back
- weak mid-back muscles.

If you enjoy crafting activities, there are numerous benefits to be gained from improving your posture: eliminating neck and back pain, strengthening weak muscles, and reducing stress on overworked muscles. Once you learn correct body mechanics, you can craft longer with more comfort.

Correct Sitting Posture

- Slide your buttocks all the way to the back of the chair seat so you are sitting squarely on your bottom. This helps spine align correctly.
- Your lower back should be right up against the lumbar support.
- Thighs should be in a ninety-degree angle to torso and lower legs in a ninety-degree angle to thigh.
- Feet should be flat on the floor. If your feet don't touch the floor, use a stool to help keep tension out of lower back.
- Arm rests should be right where your elbows naturally fall.
- Forearm should be in a ninety-degree angle, or lower, with upper arm.
- When arms rest on armrest, this takes 25 percent of the pressure off lower spinal disks and greatly decreases upper back stress.
- Sit up straight without hanging your head forward from your neck.
- Don't let upper back slump forward.

Chair Hints

- The wrong chair can cause much discomfort.
- Sitting puts 40 percent more pressure on lower back disks.
- Have a seat that is adjustable both in height and angle.
- Your chair should help keep your spine vertical, provide lumbar support, and have a swivel seat for easy shifting.

Recommended Exercises for Crafters

1. Door Frame Stretch (in chapter six)
2. Rotator Cuff Strengthener (in chapter six)

3. Wall Push-Up (in chapter four)
4. Total Posture Improvement exercises (in chapter nine)
5. Neck Glide (in chapter four)
6. Anywhere/Anytime exercises (in chapter ten)
7. Mid-back and Shoulder Strengthener (in chapter five)
8. Abdominal Strengtheners (in chapter seven)
9. The Hitchhiker (in chapter six)

Tips For Less Tension

- Take movement breaks every forty-five minutes or so.
- Work for shorter periods of time.
- During breaks, relieve muscle tensions with exercises/stretches.
- Even if doing the same craft, alternate working heights. Have one work surface that works for sitting and one that works for standing.
- Studies have linked mostly standing or mostly sitting jobs with more lower back pain than jobs where changes in posture occur.
- Get a good chair.
- Get a table that adjusts to different heights.

Chapter 17

Eating for Stronger Muscles and Bones

The foods you eat can help strengthen your muscles and bones. I'm not talking about megavitamins or exotic supplements, but good basic nutrition, with special attention to some minerals that are particularly important for good posture: potassium, magnesium, and calcium.

Healthy Choices

For good health in general, your diet should be low in saturated fats and high in lean meats (or other whole protein), whole grains, fruits, and vegetables. These foods, which reduce the risk of cancer, heart disease, and other health problems, will help your muscles and bones, too.

You also need a moderate amount of protein, which provides the building blocks for muscle tissues and bones. However, if you eat more protein than your body needs, it will just be converted into body fat. It's not true, despite the claims of protein drinks and bars, that eating lots of protein will build big muscles. According to Dr. Miriam Nelson of the School of Nutrition Science at Tufts University, our bodies rebuild and replace about one pound of muscle tissue each day. About three-quarters of the necessary protein is recycled in the process. So we need at least *one-quarter of a pound (four ounces) of protein daily* from our diet to help us maintain and repair our muscles.

According to the American Dietetic Association, between 10 and 15 percent of your calories should come from protein. For the average woman, that's about fifty grams of protein; for the average man about sixty-three grams. It's easy to get that much—two cups of skim milk, a cup of low-fat yogurt, and a small chicken breast will do it. Eat a small amount of protein with each meal.

A low-fat diet (along with regular exercise) will also help you keep your weight at a healthy level. Extra pounds put stress on the weight-bearing joints, including the spine. Extra weight in the abdominal area (an apple-shaped figure) can pull the lower back into an arch.

Potassium for Strong Muscles

For strong muscles, you need potassium, a mineral necessary for synthesizing muscle protein. The U.S. dietary goal for potassium is 2,000 milligrams per day for an average, healthy adult or child over ten. (The dietary goal for a nutrient, also called the Recommended Dietary Allowance or R.D.A., is set by the U.S. Food and Nutrition Board, National Academy of Sciences, and National Research Council.) The average American gets only 1,000 milligrams per day. Many experts agree that potassium intake from food should really be 3,500–5,000 milligrams per day.

Potassium should be derived only from food, never from a pill unless prescribed by a physician. This should not be too difficult, as it is abundant in many fruits and vegetables. You should eat between *five and nine servings of fruits and vegetables* each day.

> ### Foods High in Potassium
> Potassium is abundant in almost all fruits and vegetables. The following foods are particularly good sources of it.
> - Vegetables: asparagus, avocado, bamboo shoots, broccoli, Brussels sprouts, cauliflower, celery, endive, parsley, potatoes, rhubarb, spinach, squash, sweet potatoes, Swiss chard, tomatoes.
> - Fruits: apricots, bananas, cantaloupes, cherries, grapefruits, oranges, papayas, peaches, strawberries.
> - Dried fruits: apricots, figs, prunes, raisins.
> - Other foods: whole grains, wheat bran, wheat germ, kelp, blackstrap molasses, dairy products.

Americans come up short on potassium because we don't eat enough fruits and vegetables, and because there is way too much salt in our diet. A high-salt diet causes potassium to be lost in the urine. Processed, refined, baked, canned, and packaged foods, and frozen dinners and restaurant foods, are loaded with salt. There's salt even in chocolate milk. Potassium can also be depleted by prolonged diarrhea, stress, excessive sweating, vomiting, and the use of diuretics.

Reducing Sodium

Many people find it's easier to get more potassium in their diets than to get the sodium out. We need only 500 milligrams of sodium daily to maintain proper health, but the average American easily consumes 5,000–8,000 milligrams per day! The American Dietetic Association recommends a *maximum* of 2,400 milligrams of sodium per day, or about one teaspoon. A whopping 75 percent of all dietary salt comes from processed, packaged, and refined foods. To lower your intake:

- Check the sodium content of packaged foods by reading the labels. Many processed foods, including most canned vegetables and soups, are high in sodium. Try not to purchase foods containing added salt, sodium, or compounds like monosodium glutamate (MSG).

- When you eat in restaurants, ask for unsalted food. Send the order back if it comes salted anyway. Many restaurants now prepare low-sodium dishes. Limit fast-food meals, since they are loaded with salt.

- Experiment with lots of herbs and spices instead of using table salt in recipes.

- Many people have found fresh lemon juice to be especially helpful when trying to kick the salt habit. Lemon juice acts on the same region of your tongue that salt does—it sort of tricks your tongue into thinking it's having salt. Also, by squeezing fresh lemon juice over vegetables and meats, instead of salt, you'll be decreasing sodium and increasing vitamin C, potassium, and folic acid. Also, the vitamin C makes it easier for your body to absorb more iron from the food you are eating. Buy a few fresh lemons and keep them in your refrigerator. Cut a wedge and use as needed.

> **Foods High in Sodium**
> - Meats: bacon, bologna, canned meats, ham, hot dogs, salami, sausage.
> - Canned fish: salmon, sardines, tuna.
> - Snacks: cheeses, crackers, dips, pretzels, salted nuts.
> - Condiments: catsup, mayonnaise, mustard, olives, pickles, relish, salad dressing.
> - Seasonings: barbecue sauce, boullion cubes, celery salt, chili sauce, cooking wine, garlic salt, meat tenderizers, monosodium glutamate (MSG), onion salt, tamari sauce, smoke flavoring, soy sauce, Worchestershire sauce.

Magnesium for Muscles and Bones

While too much sodium depletes your potassium, too little magnesium does the same. Magnesium helps cells store potassium until they need it. It also aids bone growth and is necessary for the proper functioning of the nerves and muscles. In fact, magnesium is responsible for more biochemical reactions in the body than any other mineral, but unfortunately is one of the most overlooked nutrients. Make sure you get enough in your diet.

A deficiency in magnesium can cause muscle spasms or charley horses in the lower legs. If you suffer from leg spasms or muscular tension, consume several foods rich in magnesium each day. Magnesium can ease spasms within minutes of absorption.

Millions of Americans don't get enough magnesium in their diets because they don't eat enough beans, whole grains, and dark green leafy vegetables like kale, collards, and spinach. The Recommended Dietary Allowance (RDA) for magnesium is 400 milligrams for adults and 450 milligrams for pregnant, breast-feeding, or post-menopausal women. Most people don't come close. The body's supply of magnesium can be depleted by over-consumption of refined foods or high fat foods. Also, vomiting, diarrhea, use of laxatives, alcohol consumption, diet pills, diuretics, birth control pills, and even stress will cause you to lose magnesium.

If you won't eat the foods richest in magnesium, then you may need to buy a magnesium supplement. Choose one that contains magnesium citrate or magnesium malate.

Calcium for Strong Bones

Calcium is essential for strong bones. Bones store most of the body's calcium, which is also needed by the body for other purposes. Every day you do not consume enough calcium, your body will take what it needs from your bones. Day after day, week after week, year after year, and decade after decade of calcium deficiency can easily lead to osteoporosis—fragile bones.

The daily value for calcium was recently increased to 1,200 milligrams per day. During pregnancy and lactation, women need 1,200–1,500 milligrams per day. Postmenopausal women should have 1,500 milligrams of calcium daily.

The richest source of calcium is nonfat or low-fat milk and dairy products. Other sources include canned salmon with bones, tofu, broccoli, parsley, watercress, almonds, asparagus, brewer's yeast, blackstrap molasses, cabbage, carob, figs, filberts, prunes, sesame seeds, kelp, mustard greens, oats, and whole wheat.

Government statistics say that 75 percent of Americans get less than half the amount of calcium they need from their diet. That means that 75 percent of us should be taking a calcium supplement. Supplements containing calcium citrate are more easily absorbed than calcium carbonate.

Your body will probably not be able to absorb doses larger than five hundred to six hundred milligrams at a time, so split your daily dose over two or three meals. Take one of your calcium pills before bed. It is at night, when you are asleep, that your body will take calcium from your bones if there is not enough in your bloodstream. Taking a calcium supplement before bed will eliminate your body's need to take from your bones.

> **How Much Calcium Should You Supplement?**
> To figure out how many milligrams of supplement to take, start by figuring out how much calcium you usually get from food. One cup of milk or yogurt (the most common sources) contains about 300 milligrams of calcium. If you regularly have two servings, you are getting 600 milligrams a day. If you need 1,000 milligrams a day, you need 400 milligrams from supplements.

Look at the label of your calcium supplement. If it has the letters "USP," the supplement meets the U.S. Pharmacopoeia's strict standard for dissolution, and your supplement will dissolve. Try the vinegar test as well. Place one of your supplements in a cup or ordinary white vinegar and let it sit. If the supplement doesn't dissolve within thirty minutes, you may not be getting any benefit from it. Some supplements won't even dissolve if you leave them in the vinegar overnight, which means they are useless to you because they'll just pass through your digestive tract whole and the nutrients won't be available for absorption.

Vitamin D for Absorption

Vitamin D helps your body absorb calcium. Vitamin D stimulates the production of the protein carriers—boats, if you will—that carry calcium molecules through the bloodstream to their various destinations. The RDA for vitamin D is 400 international units (I.U.) a day. An eight-ounce glass of fortified milk contains one hundred units. Your body manufactures vitamin D when your skin is exposed to sunlight, but most people don't get enough of the vitamin without drinking fortified milk or taking a supplement, especially in winter when they're covered up.

Signs of a Good Supplement

It would be ideal to get all of our nutrients from fresh, healthy food, but most diets are less than ideal. If your diet isn't all it should be, a balanced, well-made multivitamin and mineral supplement can fill some of the nutritional gaps. The supplement's label should state that it contains 100 percent of the U.S. RDA (United States Recommended Dietary Allowance) for all the vitamins and minerals that the National Research Council has said are needed by the human body for health. If a product doesn't have them, don't buy it. Specifically check for:

Vitamins, Minerals, and Trace Minerals with an Established U.S. RDA	
Vitamin A	Calcium
Vitamin B1 (thiamin)	Magnesium
Vitamin B2 (riboflavin)	Boron
Vitamin B3 (niacin)	Chromium
Vitamin B5 (pantothenic acid)	Copper
Vitamin B6 (pyndoxine)	Iodine
Vitamin B12 (cobalamine)	Iron
Biotin (a B Vitamin)	Manganese
Folic acid (folate; a B vitamin)	Molybdenum
Vitamin C	Phosphorous
Vitamin D	Potassium
Vitamin E	Selenium
	Zinc

1. Similar percentages of the eight B vitamins. When one or two B vitamins are supplied in much higher amounts than others are, it throws the balance out of whack. Beware of supplements that have huge percents of the cheaper vitamins (B1, B2, B3) and much smaller amounts of others (Folic acid, B6, B12).

2. At least 100 percent RDA of biotin, a B vitamin that's vital for health. Because it is the most expensive B vitamin, many supplements have far less.

3. It should contain the following trace minerals: boron, chromium, copper, iodine, manganese, molybdenum, selenium, and zinc.

You will probably have to buy a calcium/magnesium supplement to go along with your multivitamin. Calcium and magnesium are very big molecules. If a multivitamin/mineral were to include enough of these two minerals, the tablet would be the size of a horse pill. Get calcium citrate with magnesium citrate in a ratio of two parts calcium to one part magnesium. For example, if the supplement contains 500 milligrams of calcium, it should have 250 milligrams of magnesium.

Taking supplements should never be used as an excuse to eat poorly. Look at it this way: When you eat a piece of fruit or vegetable, you get small amounts of thousands of compounds that contribute to your health. When you take a supplement, you only get a handful. Eat as well as you can—fill your diet with fruits, vegetables, grains, lean meats, nuts, and seeds and use a balanced, well-made supplement to fill in the nutritional gaps.

Fill Your Diet With High Quality, Nutrient-Dense Foods

Many people eat one or more meals each day on the run. If you know your day is going to be busy, put some healthy foods in a temperature controlled lunch bag (like some nuts, dried fruits, protein bars, yogurts, etc.) to bring with you so you are not forced, out of desperation and hunger, to grab something from a vending machine or fast food place. Fill your refrigerator and cupboards at home and at work with high quality foods as:

- Fresh fruits and veggies
- Nonfat yogurts
- Hard boiled eggs
- Healthy frozen entrees
- Nuts and seeds

- Whole grain bread and crackers
- Whole grain cereals
- Protein bars
- Salad mix and pre-cut veggies
- Canned tuna, chicken, or salmon

Phytochemicals

Phytochemicals are naturally occurring compounds found in the pigment of all fruits, vegetables, beans, and whole grains. Studies show they help just about every system in the human body function better. They also seem to be very strong anti-cancer substances.

Consume some of each color every day to get the full array of phytochemicals and all of their health contributing factors. Remember, the more brightly colored a fruit or veggie is, the more vitamins, minerals, antioxidants, and phytochemicals it contains.

Phytochemical Color Chart

Red	Orange	Yellow	Green	Blue/Purple
Tomatoes	Squashes	Corn	Spinach	Blueberries
Red Peppers	Carrots	Lemons	Broccoli	Blackberries
Beets	Apricots	Bananas	Kiwis	Plums
Strawberries	Peaches	Pineapple	Peppers	Purple Cabbage
Cherries	Cantaloupe	Grapefruit	Honeydew	Purple Grapes
Watermelon	Oranges	Pears	Avocado	Eggplant
Red Grapes	Sweet Potato	Onion	Asparagus	Boysenberries

Helpful Hint

Review your supplements to see how they stack up to government-established requirements. Replace those that fail to meet the minimum or at least add what you are lacking.

Chapter 18

Help for the New Baby Backache Blues

Good posture becomes very important when you are pregnant or have a new baby. Many common discomforts of pregnancy are linked to poor posture: an aching lower back, tight upper back, rounded shoulders, sciatic nerve pain, bladder pressure, even breathlessness. The problems don't stop after the birth—in fact, backaches become even more likely.

The weight of the baby, whether it's inside or out, puts an extra load on your spine. The mother's muscles have to support this unaccustomed load. And since the weight isn't centered over the mother's center of gravity, it can pull the alignment out of whack, especially that of the lower back. At the same time, hormones are loosening the mother's muscles and joints and making them vulnerable. No wonder the baby backache blues are so common.

During Pregnancy

During pregnancy, as at other times, lower-back pain occurs when the lower spine has an exaggerated curve. The weight of the growing baby in the uterus pulls the lower part of the spine forward into an extreme arch, causing pressure and irritation in the joints, disks, nerves, and muscles. The spine also has to support more weight than usual.

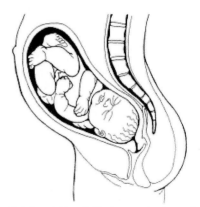

Baby's weight pulls the lower spine forward.

Most pregnant women try to compensate for the load in front by leaning their upper body back, creating even more pressure in the lower back.

During pregnancy breathing correctly can become an issue. If the upper body slumps forward because of fatigue or bad habit, lung space is decreased. As your baby grows, there is even less lung space. During pregnancy, your lungs need all the room they can get, so upper body posture becomes very important.

Slumping presses the rib cage down on the stomach, too. Like the lungs, the stomach is already short on space. It's being pressed between the growing uterus and the diaphragm. Stomach acid can be pushed into the esophagus, causing heartburn.

By standing and sitting properly, and by doing posture exercises, you can help avoid these common discomforts of pregnancy. However, it's important to stretch gently and to change or skip exercises that might put too much strain on your joints. During pregnancy and for six months afterward, you can easily injure your knees, ankles, hips, or back. All your joints are looser and less stable than usual because they're being affected by the hormones your body is producing to loosen the ligaments in the pelvis so the baby can pass through at birth. Your tendons and muscles are looser, too.

You should also skip exercises that require you to lie on your back. The American College of Obstetricians and Gynecologists (ACOG) says that women should not exercise on their backs after the fourth month of pregnancy because the heavy uterus could press on a major vein and reduce the flow of blood from the legs back to the heart. Less blood could reach your brain, causing light-headedness or dizziness. Eventually, less blood could reach the fetus. Instead, choose exercises done against a wall, standing, or sitting.

When participating in any aerobic activity, do not let your pulse rate go higher than 140 beats per minute (23 to 24 beats per ten-second count). The concern is that you'll overheat. You can sweat to lose heat but your fetus cannot, which could lead to neural tube defects during the first trimester. Never work to the point of being breathless or dripping with sweat.

Some women in the later stages of pregnancy develop carpal tunnel syndrome—numbness and tingling in their hands and fingers. If you do, skip the resistance exercises and wall push-ups.

Check with your doctor before doing this, or any other, exercise program.

If you keep these cautions in mind, you can safely and effectively improve and protect your posture during pregnancy. In fact, considering the problems poor posture can cause for you, posture improvement has never been more important than now. Here is a posture program for pregnancy:

- Practice One Minute To Better Posture in chapter three.

- To help prevent lower-back aches, do the Standing Pelvic Tilt in chapter seven.

- Remember to keep your knees soft when you're standing (stiff, locked-back knees increase the curve in your lower back).

- To stop the slump, do exercises from chapter five, and also the Shoulder Straightener and the Elbow Press in chapter six.

- To keep your abdominal muscles as strong as possible, do the Abdominal Tighteners from chapter seven often throughout the day.

- Don't do any exercises in which you lie flat on your back.

- Avoid bending from the waist. Lower your body by bending your knees and hips while keeping your back straight.

- Be mindful of how you stand, sit, move, and even sleep.

The Second Nine Months

The baby's out, so why does your back ache more than ever? During pregnancy, your abdominal muscles stretched to twice their original length. After delivery, they don't automatically shrink back. As long as the abdominals remain loose, they can't support your lower back, and it sags into an exaggerated arch that puts pressure on nerves, joints, and soft tissues.

Backaches are also caused by lifting, lowering, and carrying the baby. You're also lugging a lot of stuff around: baby, baby carrier, diaper bag, plus your purse. Your lower back really needs the support of strong abdominal muscles.

Strengthening your abs will also help you get your waistline back. During the first few months or pregnancy, the bottom three ribs flare out in anticipation of your growing baby. After you deliver, the ribs remain slightly flared unless eased back in. Since the abdominals are attached to the bottom of the rib cage, as you re-strengthen them, they will pull the ribs back in, and you'll have a waist again.

Another common postpartum problem area is the upper back. New moms spend much of their time holding, cradling, and nursing their new baby with their upper back and shoulders rounded forward. Often, they develop a lot of upper-back discomfort, including hot spots between their shoulder blades.

You can begin exercising as soon as it feels comfortable, usually after two or three weeks, but check first with your doctor.

Since you probably don't have a chunk of time to set aside for exercise, your best bets are the Anytime/Anywhere exercises (see chapter ten). Some of them can even be done while you're holding or feeding your baby.

Be sure to do the exercises that strengthen your abdominal muscles-only the sitting ones. Next, focus on stopping the slump. Practice the One Minute To Better Posture technique in chapter three as well as the sitting and standing exercises in the chapters four, five, and six. Do stretches carefully and moderately, since your ligaments can remain loose for up to six months after the birth. Don't be discouraged if the results aren't immediate. It took nine months for your body to get this way.

How to Lift a Baby

To protect your back, pay attention to the position of your body when you are feeding, changing, and carrying your baby. The new father should use safe lifting techniques, too.

Carrying your baby

Many mothers and fathers lean back to compensate for the child's weight. This puts pressure on the lower back and results in pain and discomfort. When holding or carrying your baby, make sure your hips are tucked under, abdominals pulled in, and torso held erect. Avoid always carrying your baby on the same side. Switch sides often, or try to carry your baby in front so the weight is evenly distributed. Baby backpacks center the weight evenly across your back, but be sure not to tip your torso back or too far forward to compensate for the extra weight you're carrying. Snugglies allow you to carry your baby in front, evenly centered. Your baby can hear your heartbeat and be within your sight, too. Some slings can put too much pressure on one shoulder, but others, I've been told, are really comfortable. There are many different kinds of baby-carrying devices on the market—try them out, if possible, in the store before buying one.

Baths

For the first six months, bathe your baby in the kitchen sink rather than bending over a tub. (While you're standing there, you can work in a Pelvic Tilt, Abdomen Tightener, or Buttock Clencher.)

Feeding

When breast-feeding or bottle-feeding, instead of rounding your upper back forward to reach the baby, bring the baby up to you. If you're breast-feeding, turn the baby completely toward you (you'll be tummy to tummy). Rest the baby's weight on some pillows in your lap, rather than fully in your arms.

Car seats

Car seats are safe for babies, but treacherous for their parents' backs. When you put the baby in a car seat, you have to twist your torso and hold the baby's full weight with your arms stretched out. This puts a tremendous strain on the disks and ligaments in your back. To reduce the strain, reduce the distance you have to reach. To place an infant in a rear-facing car seat, sit on the seat next to the car seat, then place the infant in the chair. To put a child in a forward-facing seat, first tighten your abdominals to support your back, then get as close to the car seat as possible. While facing the rear of the car, place your foot inside on the rear floor so most of your body is inside the car. You should be squatting slightly, and your torso should not be twisted.

Cribs

Putting your baby into and out of a crib can be hazardous to your back if you don't lift and bend with caution. Remember that for the first six months after delivery, your back is vulnerable because your ligaments are still loose and your abdominals are still stretched. Raise the crib mattress to the highest level for the first six months so you don't have to lean over so far. Before lifting your baby, always support your back by tightening your abdominal muscles and keeping your pelvis in neutral. Keep your knees slightly bent as you lift. Avoid twisting your back when lifting the baby up or placing the baby back down.

Congratulations on your new family addition. I'm sure you've found by now that you love this child as you have loved nothing else on this earth. All the physical stress and strain pales in comparison to the new life in your midst. Keep in mind that your body can spring back to pre-pregnancy strength. Keep working on strengthening all four layers of abdominal muscles and on using good body mechanics. Keeping your back and joints healthy and pain free will help you enjoy this experience fully.

Chapter 19

Osteoporosis and Posture

The term osteoporosis literally means porous bones. If bones have lost density, you are more prone to fractures and breaks.

Bone Basics

- Twenty-five million Americans have osteoporosis.

- Thirty-four million have bone density low enough to increase their risk of fractures.

- Half of women over sixty-five have osteoporosis.

- Eighteen percent of women age twenty-five to thirty-four already have low bone density.

- Fifty percent of postmenopausal women will break a bone as a result of low bone density.

The only way to know your bone density is to have a bone density scan. Ask your doctor for a referral. The sooner you get a bone density scan, the better. If for no other reason you'll have a baseline to compare against as you age.

Low bone density can cause bones to fracture easily. These fractures, most often in the wrist, hip, or spine, are not only painful, but can limit a woman's activities and independence.

Osteoporosis affects men also. But men start out with thicker bones than women so it takes them longer to be in danger of fracturing, usually not until around the age of eighty. However, men also need to consume adequate calcium to keep themselves healthy.

Though the effects of osteoporosis are seen in older people, mostly women, the condition develops over a lifetime. People of every age can build stronger bones to help avoid this. In this chapter, you'll learn ways to help increase your bone density. If you have already been diagnosed with osteoporosis, you'll learn how to reduce your risk of fractures by improving your posture and muscle strength. If you have low bone density, working on improving posture is crucial, for it can stop the rounding over and height loss that occurs. It will help prevent pressure on spinal bones and help prevent fractures.

Building Stronger Bones

Though bones look like permanent structures, their tissues are constantly being removed and added. Until a person is about twenty-five, new bone cells are added faster than old bone cells are removed, so the bones become larger and denser. After thirty-five, bone is lost faster than it's added, particularly after menopause—unless the person takes steps to build bone. Decades of research shows there is a lot you can do not only to slow bone loss, but actually increase bone density after the age of thirty-five.

There are three ways to keep your bones strong: diet, weight-bearing exercise, and strengthening exercise.

Nutrition

At every age, calcium is essential for strong bones, because it increases the density of the bones. Your body also needs calcium for other functions, including the contraction of the heart and other muscles. Every day that you do not consume enough calcium in your diet, your body has no choice but to take calcium from your bones to meet its needs and your bones become weaker and weaker year after year.

Calcium is the mineral that fills in your bones and makes them dense. Magnesium is the mineral that makes the underlying structure of bone–the bone matrix–strong. You need calcium for dense bones and magnesium for strong bones.

Calcium, magnesium, and vitamin D requirements and sources are covered extensively in chapter seventeen.

Avoid drinking pop or too much caffeine containing beverages. For every cup of caffeinated beverages you drink, you use up forty milligrams of calcium. For every four-ounce piece of meat (about the size of a deck of cards) eaten you lose about one hundred milligrams of your calcium to neutralize the acid created.

Weight-Bearing Exercise

To build your bones, you have to do activities that put weight on them. Walking, jogging, and weight lifting are good examples. Just as your heart and lungs become stronger with regular aerobic exercise, your bones become stronger with regular weight-bearing exercise. Research done at the University of Minnesota shows that three hours of weight-bearing exercise each week can decrease bone loss by 75 percent. Exercise can even increase bone mass after menopause. No matter what your age, it is never too late to benefit from exercise.

Make weight-bearing exercise a regular part of your life. Walking is excellent for overall health and well-being. Join a walking club or enlist a neighbor to walk with you regularly. To start, walk for ten or fifteen minutes. Gradually lengthen the walk to thirty to forty-five minutes or longer.

Strengthening Exercise

Strengthening exercise is extremely important and can greatly impact bone density. Every time you contract a muscle, the tendon pulls on the bone. This sends signals to the brain to send minerals to that bone to strengthen it.

If You Have Osteoporosis

If you have been diagnosed with osteoporosis, your risk of bone fractures is very high, so you should check with your doctor or physical therapist before you embark on an exercise program to ensure that you don't put too much stress on your bones.

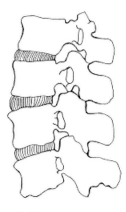

Healthy vertebrae

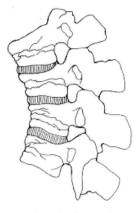

Vertebrae that have collapsed

If you get the go-ahead, exercises that improve the flexibility and strength of your back can help relieve the pain of spinal fractures and reduce the chances that more will occur. When the bones have been weakened by osteoporosis, hairline cracks can occur in the vertebrae that make up the spine. Eventually, the body's weight can crush the weakened vertebra. These painful fractures cause tremendous curving of the upper spine and loss of height.

A slouched, rounded-forward posture increases the chance that a vertebra will fracture and collapse, because it puts stress on the area most likely to fracture. All of the tips, techniques, and exercises included in this book will help you stop the rounding over that occurs as you age, and will help take pressure off spinal bones.

Regularly practice the One Minute To Better Posture technique. Every time you think of it, lift your rib cage, pull your shoulder blades back, and pull your belly muscles in. Also, be sure to do the Abdominal Tighteners in chapter seven. Concentrating on the breathing portion of the exercises. They will help keep your rib cage joints functional.

By increasing the strength of your legs and the flexibility of your ankles, you'll reduce your risk of falls. Many fractures happen because older people lose their balance easily (even when making an ordinary move like turning too fast or reaching up or down), then don't have the strength to stop themselves once they start to topple. Try the strengthening exercises for your feet and ankles. They'll also improve ankle flexibility.

For all of the exercises, start with three repetitions and gradually build to ten, adding one each day. If any exercise causes discomfort, omit it. For the resistance exercises, try one repetition and see how your joints feel. Choose the easier versions of exercises and always use very light resistance to begin.

Fall-Proof Your Home

- Secure all rugs to the floor. Get rid of all scatter rugs. Don't use floor polish, which makes floors too slippery.
- Keep the floors clear of clutter.
- Make sure phone and electrical cords are out of the way.
- Light the hallways, closets, and stairwells.
- Keep a flashlight by your bed.
- Install grab bars in your tub and near your toilet. Buy a good non-slip bath mat, too.
- On stairs, secure carpets well and add treads if possible. Use the banister.
- Work on increasing your leg strength and ankle flexibility.
- Wear shoes with rubber or non-slip soles.

Don't do exercises in which you would bend forward at the waist or twist your spine—there aren't any in this book, but you may encounter them in other exercise programs or classes.

All of the lying down exercises should be done on your bed, because getting down to and up from the floor could be too difficult. If your upper back is too curved forward, you may need to place a thin pillow under your head so your neck doesn't have to arch in order for your head to rest against the bed.

Helpful Hint

Proper lifting and other good body mechanics become even more important if you have osteoporosis. To protect your back:

- Never bend over to pick up an object. This places too much pressure on the front of the vertebrae and can lead to compression fractures of the spine.

- After brushing your teeth, spit into the sink by bending at the knees rather than the waist.

- When coughing or sneezing, place one hand on your lower back, lift your rib cage up, and tighten your abdominals. This will help protect vertebrae and disks from injury caused by a sudden bend forward.

- Never bend or twist the spine when vacuuming or raking.

- Don't sit too long. While sitting, circle your ankles in different directions.

- When you need to stand in place for more than a few minutes, put one of your feet up on a stool or railing.

- Try to stay as active as possible. Inactivity causes bones to weaken further.

When Should You Seek Medical Help?

Research shows that 90 percent of back problems eventually resolve and heal themselves without medical intervention and that most people resume normal activities within a month. However, if you have back or neck pain that occurs suddenly, or that has lasted a long time, seek medical help.

Usually, sudden pain follows years of poor posture, when the person bends, lifts, or reaches. Improving posture and body mechanics (the way one sits, stands, moves, lifts) is the best way to prevent a recurrence.

Treating Minor Pain Yourself

If you have a minor backache or neck ache, your goal is to reduce the pain and inflammation. Inflammation stretches the tissues, causing more pain and interfering with healing.

- Take an anti-inflammatory pain reliever like aspirin (unless you are allergic to it) or ibuprofen. These over-the-counter drugs are just as effective as prescription muscle relaxants and have few side effects.

- As soon as possible after an injury, ice it down. Keep icing it for ten to twenty minutes every two hours for forty-eight hours or until the swelling subsides. You can use a frozen blue gel pack, or place ice cubes in a plastic bag, or use a bag of frozen corn kernels or peas. Wrap either in a thin towel—never apply directly to the skin.

- Rest, but only for the first day. A Finnish study published in the *New England Journal of Medicine* showed that even two days of bed rest can slow recovery by weakening the muscles. Try to go about your normal activities.

When to Seek Medical Care

You should see your doctor if you have back or neck pain and:

- You have been in an accident (a car accident or a fall).

- You feel numbness or tingling.

- There is a line of shooting pain into your buttocks or legs.

- The pain is sharp or stabbing.

- There is stiffness or a decrease in range of motion.

- You have any weakness in your ankle, big toe, hand, or fingers, or a loss of gripping power in your hand.

- A neck pain persists longer than ten days, or a stiff neck is accompanied by fever or nausea (symptoms of meningitis).

Conventional medical treatment will start with an examination by your primary care physician. The doctor will evaluate the pain and will want to rule out any serious problems, such as fracture, dislocation, or tumor. You may have imaging studies such as an x-ray, CT scan, or MRI to detect bone or soft tissue damage.

You may be referred to a specialist. If nerve damage is suspected, you'll be referred to a neurologist (a medical doctor who treats disorders of the brain, spine, and nerves) or a neurosurgeon. Orthopedists and orthopedic surgeons specialize in bones, joints, and muscles. They treat a wide range of problems, from herniated disks to traumatic injuries.

If it is suspected you have injured a muscle or joint, your doctor may refer you to a registered licensed physical therapist. Look for a therapist who specializes in back and neck pain. The therapist will evaluate your posture and the source of your pain, then teach you specific exercises and stretches for your individual needs. The therapist will also show you ways to move through your daily activities as efficiently as possible while protecting your back.

Alternative Therapies

A wide range of alternative therapies places great importance on posture. You may find one of them will help you develop better posture as well as relieve pain in your back, neck, or elsewhere. When pursuing an alternative therapy, look for a practitioner who has been trained and licensed. Tell your medical doctor that you plan to try the alternative therapy.

Chiropractic Care

Chiropractors, also know as doctors of chiropractic or chiropractic physicians, diagnose and treat problems associated with the body's muscular, nervous and skeletal systems, especially the spine. Chiropractors hold that vertebral misalignments not only cause pain, but alter many important body junctions by affecting the nervous system. Chiropractors take into account the patient's overall health and wellness. Many work with exercise, diet, and lifestyle counseling, in addition to spinal manipulation, also known as chiropractic adjustments. Adjustments of the affected joint and tissues can restore mobility, alleviate pain and muscle tightness, and allow tissues to heal.

Physical Therapy

Physical therapists examine, evaluate and treat people recovering from injury or surgery and disease. They have extensive education in anatomy and body mechanics. They work to correct postural imbalances, increase muscle strength and endurance. They seek to restore joint range of motion, coordination, and decrease muscle and joint pain. They use a wide range of non-invasive interventions, like therapeutic exercise, massage, heat, cold, ultrasound, hydrotherapy, and electrical stimulation, to reduce pain and restore function for individuals dealing with injury, disability or disease. Physical therapists also help people prevent injury or recurrence of injury. In most cases, a doctor's referral is needed to see a physical therapist.

Bodywork

Many alternative therapies and techniques can relieve the tension and stress in muscles. The Alexander Technique teaches people to properly align the head, neck, and torso, and consciously use new and better patterns of movement. Yoga is a wonderful way to increase flexibility (but avoid poses that arch the neck and lower back: for example, the plough). There are massage therapies like Swedish massage as well as deep tissue manipulation like Rolfing. You may wish to explore some of these therapies.

Acupuncture

Acupuncture has been used as a healing art in China for over three thousand years. The principle behind acupuncture is to balance the body's flow of energy. If the acupuncturist finds an imbalance of energy flow, he or she will place very thin sterile needles into specific meridian points. Acupuncturists believe pain is caused by a block in energy. The fine needles restore the flow.

Most people feel nothing when the needles are inserted just below the skin. Some feel a slight sensation. Although they may sound frightening, acupuncture treatments are not painful. Most people find them comforting and relaxing. And many have found relief from aches and pains.

Make sure the acupuncturist you choose has proper credentials and that they are either a Certified Acupuncturist (C.A.) or a Licensed Acupuncturist (L.Ac.).

Exercises and Stretches

About the Author

Janice Novak developed her unique posture program over twenty years of working with individual clients and teaching thousands of workshops for hospitals, universities, and professional organizations. She holds a master's degree in health and physical education, and has been quoted in many national magazines such as *Ladies Home Journal, Woman's Day, Muscle & Fitness, Natural Health,* and *American Baby* to name a few. Janice regularly presents health segments for television and radio, including an appearance on the Oprah Winfrey Show discussing her book, *Posture, Get It Straight.*